THE EDGE OF STRENGTH

An Unconventional Guide to Live Your Strength
&
Discover Your Greatness

By Scott Iardella,
MPT, CSCS, CISSN, SFGII, SFL, FMS, USAW, Pn1

The Edge of Strength

An Unconventional Guide to
Live Your Strength
&
Discover Your Greatness

By Scott Iardella,
MPT, CSCS, CISSN, SFGII, SFL, FMS, USAW, Pn1

1st edition 2015

Library of Congress Control Number:

Printed in the United States of America

ISBN Paperback: 978-0692577110

Edited by Dominique Chatterjee

Cover Design by elementi-studio.com

Cover Photo by Ann Remotigue Photography

Design, Layout, and Typesetting by Alexander Becker
www.alexanderbecker.net

DEDICATION

The Edge of Strength is dedicated to my beautiful and amazing wife, Tanya, for her patience, understanding, and strong support throughout the book writing process. She is truly the strength for our family and without her, this book would not have been possible.

I also dedicate this book to our little girls, Alexis and Ava. You are the driving force in my life. I hope that this book will be an inspiration for you to live a strong, successful life in everything that you do. Because of you, I am committed to being forever strong.

"Life is hard if you live it the easy way
and it's easy if you live it the hard way."
–Unknown

If you apply the philosophy, methods, principles, and techniques in this book...

YOUR LIFE WILL BE EASY.

Table of Contents

DISCLAIMER

This book is for general information purposes only. Individuals should always be medically cleared for any exercise or nutritional modifications by their health care provider, before initiating any advice or recommendations provided in *The Edge of Strength*.

This book is not a substitute for professional medical advice or to treat any specific disorders or medical conditions. Any action or application of material presented in *The Edge of Strength* is at the reader's discretion and is the sole responsibility of the individual.

The author, publisher, and all parties involved in the production of *The Edge of Strength* assume no liability whatsoever.

This book is for everyone who wants more out of life.

It's not mainstream.

It's not filled with shortcuts or quick fixes.

It's not hype.

It's not the latest fitness fad or trend.

It is what works.

If you share any of the values below, then this book is for you.

- Achievement
- Boldness
- Determination
- Excellence
- Focus
- Freedom
- Fulfillment
- Growth
- Health
- Learning
- Persistence
- Personal Mastery
- Simplicity
- Strength
- Victory

I hope that by reading this book, it will help you take control and get mind-blowing health and fitness results over the long term.

There is something for you in the pages ahead.

A SIMPLE MISSION

Hey, I'm Scott. I've got a simple mission.

To help people of all levels live their strength and discover their greatness through a foundation of strength.

It's that simple.

I created RdellaTraining.com to help support that mission.

I'm privileged to have unique experiences as an athlete, strength coach, and physical therapist that have taught me how to apply the science and practice of human movement and performance to maximize results and minimize injury.

I help people train safer, stronger, and smarter to improve their physical potential using proven methods such as bodyweight training, kettlebells, and barbells, among other things.

I don't just talk theory. I live it.

This book represents everything I'm passionate about and condenses much of what I've discovered through 3 decades of training.

I've had my share of struggles and setbacks, but I have viewed those as opportunities to learn and grow.

You and I have limitless physical potential regardless of age, gender, or background. You need to believe that.

This book will help move you closer to uncovering that potential.

The Edge of Strength will help you discover your strength or advance it to a higher level.

This book is for the serious fitness enthusiast, the intelligent lifter, the coach, and the everyday athlete.

If you're a novice, you'll gain practical knowledge, learn how to apply it in action, and understand how to keep yourself motivated along the way.

If you're more advanced, you need every available edge to continue to make progress. There's a wealth of information available in this book, so you're bound to stumble on a new technique or mindset to reach the next level.

My intention is to keep things simple, to take complex ideas and simplify to only what is essential.

The information presented in the pages ahead comes directly from:

- Decades of unique experiences as a physical therapist, coach, and athlete;
- Countless books I've read on related subject matter;
- Personal notes from numerous workshops and seminars I've attended; and
- Key insights from personal conversations with some of the most brilliant minds in the industry – renowned experts such as Pavel Tsatsouline, Dan John, Gray Cook, Kelly Starrett, Dr. Fred Hatfield, Greg Everett, Charlie Weingroff, and so many more great coaches and fitness professionals than I could name.

I'm excited for you to take this journey toward gaining new strength.

Let's do this.

This book is for everyone who wants to become the best version of themselves for the rest of their lives.

*"What a disgrace it is for a man to grow old
without ever seeing the beauty and strength
of which his body is capable."*
–Socrates

INTRODUCTION

Begin with end in mind.
—Steven Covey

At the lowest point of my life, I was weak, immobile, and couldn't get out of pain.

I was suffering.

Actually, it was hell.

My muscles deteriorated, I couldn't sleep, I couldn't function, I lost strength every day, and it was the most helpless situation I've ever experienced.

I literally couldn't even stand upright due the excruciating pain from sciatic scoliosis.

My body and my physical state were a complete mess.

It was the darkest of times.

And I was 19 years old.

That experience changed my life forever. Ultimately, that experience led to the writing of this book. This is why I'm so passionate and believe that anyone can benefit from gaining strength.

The Edge of Strength is about taking control of your body and your health to be the best version of yourself.

You can ignore the information in this book, but that may leave you in the same spot you're in right now or worse.

I want you to move forward, not regress or settle for status quo. That's the worst place to be and no one deserves to settle for average or mediocre.

I want you to discover your inherent greatness.

How is what you're doing working for you? Or more to the point, how is what you're doing not working for you?

If you're like most people, there are still challenges you want to overcome:

- Not performing at the level you expect
- Missing workouts or lacking consistency
- Dealing with injuries or joint mobility issues
- Feeling the frustration about not losing body fat
- Dealing with slow gains or lack of progress

- Experiencing destructive mental blocks like self-doubt, procrastination, and impatience

By understanding a simple foundation of **training fundamentals,** you can better tackle these challenges now and into the future.

Physical strength is the one thing in your control that helps every facet of life and generally improves quality of living. **Strength is our fountain of youth.**

On the flip side, not having strength can be limiting, debilitating, and make us weak in so many ways.

REVOLUTION STRONG

*"We need to spend less time on what we can't be
and spend more time on what we can be."*
–Gary Vaynerchuk

There's a new revolution.

This book is about achieving your physical potential, no matter who you are or how far along you are in the journey.

Regardless of age, gender, ability, or background – you have the capacity to become stronger.

We're living in exciting times today because men and women all over the world are discovering that we have unbelievable physical potential. Physical strength and the qualities of strength are the unbeatable edge – not just in terms of sport performance – but in life.

Stronger people can battle through more. They are better equipped to handle the everyday challenges that life throws at them. They are part of the new revolution today I call **"Revolution Strong."**

But the revolution has a few problems.

- Extreme workouts.
- Irrational training.
- The lure of shortcuts and quick fixes.

Myths, misinformation, and pure lack of understanding are problems in today's fitness climate. Let's look at the common trend of "extreme" workouts as an example. Extreme workouts are beyond high-intensity – past your breaking point.

They're designed to smash you.

These extremists believe that in order to have a good workout, you have to feel trashed after the session; otherwise, it wasn't a "good workout" in their opinion. Somehow, there is a misconception that after a workout you need to be drenched in a pool of sweat and sprawled out across the floor in complete exhaustion.

Continuous overexertion is no way to approach training for the long term. Extreme workouts are based on faulty thinking and I'll explain why in this book.

THE EDGE

The major goal in this book is to provide a **rational approach** to strength and performance training to achieve extraordinary health and fitness results throughout the rest of your life.

It's a book about the **process of mastery** and the road to **continuous improvement.**

This is not a short-term approach, but a sustainable solution to ultimate health and performance.

There is only one prerequisite to the material in this book, and it's important. I assume if you're reading this, you want to be stronger. But **you must also have the DESIRE to improve.**

If you have desire to unleash your physical potential, then this book will help you gain *The Edge of Strength.*

It's not for the dabbler, the person looking for the latest way to lose weight. This guide is for every person who is committed to learning more about how to optimize their physical potential, whether you're starting as a fitness novice or an advanced athlete.

As you read the book, there's one thing I ask from you.

Reject that voice in your head when you're reading that says,

"Yeah, I already know this."

If you know this, then are you doing these techniques, are you implementing these strategies every day, and are you living your strength?

Be open to learning and further reinforcing your knowledge.

We are all students.

The goal isn't to push one single tool or method of gaining strength, but help you fill in the gaps to get to the next level.

THE PROMISE OF THIS BOOK

I want to share with you the **strength training system and approach** that radically and dramatically changed my life. The information shared in this book have given me:

- The highest levels of health and energy
- A level of strength and physical performance that I'd never before experienced (even compared to my 20s!)
- Improved body composition: more muscle, less fat
- A renewed sense of purpose with my long-term training approach
- An amazing new level of mobility, flexibility, and resiliency

And, I know it can do the same for you.

When I changed my training, it provided these benefits even after decades of training experience and overcoming a major injury.

I train harder, smarter, and better – and you can too.

In short, I've literally become **the strongest version** of myself by implementing these strategies and methods.

The Edge of Strength is for anyone who wants to become stronger not only physically, but mentally, emotionally, socially, spiritually, and in every way possible.

You'll learn how to:

- Define your most important goals
- Hit new personal records in your lifts
- Add lean, quality muscle over 6-12 weeks
- Dramatically improve your body composition
- Move more supple, mobile, and strong
- Maximize your training results and surpass hurdles
- Minimize the risk for injury
- Feel powerful, more energetic, and more confident in life

This might sound like an exaggeration, but remember it's about the long haul, not a quick fix.

If you're interested in improving any or all of these things, if you're committed to improving your life, it's time to get started.

Are you ready to join Revolution Strong?

SECTION I – DEFINING STRENGTH

*"The strongest people are not those who show strength in front of us –
but those who win battles we know nothing about."*
–Unknown

CHAPTER 1: A FOUNDATION OF STRENGTH

"It's NEVER to late to become what you might have been."
–George Eliot

Strength is all about the approach, so let's start by taking a look at how to approach *The Edge of Strength* concepts.

Applying the fundamental concepts in this book will help you achieve results more effectively over the long term, and you'll be able to do so as safely as possible.

While I definitely advocate heavy lifting, you must do this as safely and as strategically as possible. This is extremely important to understand in a fitness climate where there's so much irrational advice and misinformation.

Nothing has really changed in fitness through the years, although new fads and gimmicks come and go all the time. **Strength and performance are all about the fundamentals,** and it always has been.

Squat, deadlift, press, and lift heavy things. Learn to move better. Get up and down from the ground. Simple movements are what work. But, simple does NOT mean easy.

If you apply the principles and ideas in this book, you will come away with transformational concepts that will make a major difference, not only in your physical training, performance, and physical self but in your life.

Strength is life, and life is strength.

IMAGINE

Imagine being truly happy with yourself because you feel so healthy, alive, and strong.

Imagine yourself as a high-performing, powerful machine in your everyday life.

If you begin to think of your body this way, you'll respect it and have a greater appreciation for your abilities.

You'll respect how you treat your body, what you put into it, and how you approach your training.

It all starts by thinking differently.

If you can make this simple shift in thinking, I guarantee it will make a difference.

There's NOTHING like feeling strong.

I heard a powerful statement recently.

"Common sense is not always common practice."

This book is a standard for common practice. That means that I hope you put this information into your daily practice.

WHAT CAN STRENGTH DO FOR YOU?

Here's a specific example.

"For quite some time throughout my life, I felt I didn't have enough confidence to succeed. It showed in how I walked, as I was always the tall Asian girl, towering over the guys in school.

When I started kettlebell training 3 years ago, those insecurities came out and I struggled to overcome them. It wasn't until the last few months when a new program and coach changed my outlook. Working with barbell deadlifts really empowered me and it also carried over into my kettlebell lifts.

I found myself able to take on what challenges life brought me. I never considered how this changed my presence, until one coach mentioned how he noticed the change since he saw me last year.

How you feel about yourself will ultimately translate to how your body responds. It's pretty powerful. Respect it."

–Suzanne Ko

Strength can have a profound effect in our lives as you just read. There's so many great stories like Suzanne's.

Strength means many different things to people, and there are many different qualities of strength (which you'll learn about).

- What does strength mean to you?
- How do you define strength?

These are some questions to consider as we begin.

This book is a blueprint from going where you are right now (Point A) to where you want to be (Point B).

If you understand and apply the **principles** and **fundamentals,** you can produce great results for a long time to come.

But, **it's only valuable if you take action with the information.**

Many "fitness books" make claims about body transformation and that's all well and good.

It's great to achieve body transformation, but this book is about life transformation.

I want you to truly understand the importance of improving, developing, and maintaining the qualities of strength.

The health and performance consequences of lack of strength is literally quite devastating – ranging from the increased incidence of major life-threatening diseases to a significant functional decline leading to increased mortality.

Lack of strength can literally kill us – I'll show you the research to prove it.

We'll cover the devastating science on strength loss in more detail later (Chapter 6).

OVERVIEW

In Section I (Understanding Strength), we cover the background you'll need to understand about why strength training is so important for health and performance.

In Section II, (Approaching Strength), we cover important laws, rules, and insights of successful strength training for the long term.

In Section III, (Planning for Strength) we cover key habits, mindsets, nutrition, and how to develop laser focus.

And, finally in Section IV, (Developing Strength) we'll cover the "how to" with the specific methods and techniques I've used that make the biggest difference.

I'll show you how to take action with this material and apply what's most relevant to you.

The Edge of Strength is a philosophy and methodology of high-level performance.

Throughout the book, we'll focus on 5 areas of physical development:

- **Human Movement**
- **Bodyweight Training**
- **Kettlebell Training**

- **Powerlifting**
- **Olympic Weightlifting**

It's no secret that these proven methods have been used by countless athletes and fitness enthusiasts all over the world.

These are the methods that I have found to be most valuable to provide the foundation of strength. This isn't to say this is all you should do. But, this is what I focus on and will continue to do for many years ahead, even as a man in my 40s.

No matter how you achieve it, there is almost nothing greater for human health and performance than training for strength.

Refuse ordinary, and get the edge.

Strength is your edge.

CHAPTER 2: STRENGTH IS YOUR EDGE

"Everything you want lies outside of your comfort zone."
–Keith Cunningham

A fighter needs to be highly conditioned.

A highly conditioned fighter will defeat a de-conditioned fighter every day of the week. But if conditioning is equal, the stronger fighter will ALWAYS be the better fighter.

No matter what the sport, the stronger athlete is the better athlete when all else is equal.

Building a foundation of strength makes every other physical quality better.

Strength is the edge.

It's the edge in life.

It's the edge in sport.

Strength is the ONE physical quality that improves every aspect of performance.

The good news is you are MUCH stronger than you can possibly imagine.

And strength is more important than you can imagine.

Just read the great work of Earle Liederman, George Hackenschmidt, or Arthur Saxon who wrote about the obvious benefits of strength so many years ago.

These strength legends paved the way for where we are today.

We should train hard and take it to the edge, but never over the edge.

Over-the-edge training is reckless and dangerous.

We have to **be rational** to keep injury prevention in the forefront of our training objectives.

And, despite conventional thinking, strength training is extremely safe when done with **proper technique** and with **intelligent programming strategies,** which I'll reinforce throughout this book.

One of the major problems in the fitness industry is that most people do not understand the importance of physical strength and what it means for total health, performance, and body composition.

After reading this, you'll know WHY to be strong and HOW to be strong.

You were meant to be strong.

You are designed to be strong.

Physical strength is your best strategy for a healthy, high-performing, resilient life.

No matter what physical level you are at right now, you can forge a stronger, more mobile, supple, and more athletic body that you can improve for the rest of your life.

Here's the undeniable "edge" that strength can enhance for each of us:

- muscle mass (hypertrophy)
- joint mobility
- flexibility
- conditioning
- functional movement skills
- stronger bones, joints, and connective tissue
- explosive power
- improved athletic performance
- mental toughness
- cardiovascular benefits (program dependent)
- muscular endurance
- speed
- coordination
- balance
- improved neuromuscular efficiency
- suppleness
- body composition changes (more muscle, less fat)
- stamina
- improved technical skills
- prevention of muscle tissue loss (sarcopenia)
- optimizing hormonal function
- spinal strength and stability
- prevention of disease and functional decline
- prevention of illness

- gross motor skill development
- improved confidence, self-esteem, and sense of wellbeing
- resiliency
- improved cognitive function

This list speaks volumes about the benefits of being stronger. We can choose to be strong, or we will eventually suffer the consequences.

Before we move forward, I want you to know that **strength is NOT the only thing we need.** I'll cover all the other important physical qualities later – **endurance, speed, flexibility** – the difference being that strength is foundational.

The extent and quality of strength will depend on the training goal.

THE FOUNDATION FOR A BETTER LIFE

When I started training over 30 years ago, I didn't know the first thing about strength or performance.

I was just trying to put on muscle as a "bodybuilder." Every young kid who starts out lifting weights wants to impress with a strong, muscular, powerful physique.

Muscle is very important as well (we'll get into that later).

But, what I've discovered through the years is that strength is vital, and it depends on more than muscles. No matter what your goals are, strength matters.

Forever Strong is a simple mantra we should all live by for the rest of our lives, yet most of us don't. The longer you can continue to lift heavy things, the less likely your chances to become weak, de-conditioned, and non-functional.

Every single day, we get a day older.

And, guess what we lose?

Physical strength.

Every day, we get a little bit weaker, unless we proactively do something about it.

We can't stop the aging process, but we can do things to negate the effects. Do you realize there are 80-year-old competitive Olympic weightlifter athletes in this world? That blows my mind! It demonstrates that nothing is impossible.

My goal is to help you understand the importance of physical strength – and not just for the sake of getting stronger but to optimize your entire life.

Not only is it my job to help you understand that, but I'll show you why strength is the key to unlocking your potential and getting the health and fitness results you want. I'll even show you **how strong is strong enough** to reach your goals and maintain a high level of performance.

We lose strength and other qualities such as mobility, muscle mass, cardiovascular capacity (Vo2 max), and movement skills – unless we do the right things to negate the losses.

We must not only preserve our strength but build on it one day at a time.

MOVEMENT PRECEDES STRENGTH

"Movement is our vital sign."
–Gray Cook

Before strength, we need to have a baseline of quality movement.

To move well, you need to have mobility and stability before moving strong. This is part of what I call safe strength. We'll discuss movement in greater detail in Chapter 7.

Unlike many fitness books which list countless exercises, I'm going to cover **the vital few that elicit superior results.** I'll share tips to improve movement, mobility, and stability with the key exercises I cover.

The stronger you are physically, the stronger you are in life. And studies prove this.

No matter who you are or where you are in the process, you can maximize your potential by becoming the best version of yourself, the strongest version of yourself by gaining *The Edge of Strength*.

THE 1% RULE

I've been living by the 1% rule now for a while, but I didn't realize it. This powerful concept caught my attention thanks to James Altucher, an entrepreneur, writer, and podcaster.

He's not a strength athlete, coach, or anything like that, but his point on the 1% rule is spot on. And, it ties into the philosophy of this book and my message to you.

Focus on progress for the rest of your life – no matter what your age, background, or training status is.

I realize we get older and things change, but why would we ever stop trying to improve ourselves? Progress is about moving forward in some way every day.

Be better tomorrow than you were today. That is *The Edge of Strength* philosophy.

Frankly, **maintenance is almost regression.** Although it means you aren't getting worse, you're also not getting better.

You didn't wake up today to be mediocre, average, or status quo.

The 1% rule is to strive to get better every day by just 1%. Framing progress in this way helps us focus on continuous improvement without getting overwhelmed.

Each training session, each day in some way, make yourself better by a mere 1%.

Improve your nutrition, improve your thinking, help others, develop yourself, lift better, learn something new.

How do you measure the 1% rule?

All it takes is a little awareness. At the end of every day, ask yourself how you improved. Where did you get a little better today?

That's all this is: retooling your mindset to focus on what you're doing right and how you can keep that progress going tomorrow.

The 1% rule is a game changer.

CHAPTER 3: IMPORTANT TERMS AND CONCEPTS

"Strength is a Skill."
–Pavel Tsatsouline

This chapter lays the groundwork with some important training terms and concepts. You're going to learn the language of strength and performance.

I'd recommend reading this through so you have the essential background you need and understand the material moving forward in the book. Then you may want to continue to refer back to this as you need to.

STRENGTH

First, we have to understand what strength means, and the truth is that it can be very general term.

When we say strength, we need to know the kind of strength we're talking about. We also have to be clear on understanding the different types or qualities of strength, which are covered in the next chapter.

So, what is strength?

Strength is the ability to generate force.

More specifically, it's the ability of a particular group of muscles to generate force under certain conditions.

Strength = Ability to Generate Force

POWER

Power is the ability to generate force quickly.

This is an important quality in strength and athletic development.

We will all want to develop the quality of power for a lifetime and I'll discuss why in Chapter 6.

The quality of power isn't just for athletes, but for everyone.

MUSCLE ACTIONS

Isometric: Muscle gains tension, but no change in length

Concentric: Muscle gains tension and shortens

Eccentric: Muscle gains tension and lengthens

Plyometric: Concentric preceded by eccentric

ONE REP MAX (1 RM)

The 1 RM is the common indicator for maximum strength for a given exercise. If you can lift 300 pounds on the bench press for one repetition with good technique, that's your 1 RM.

A 1 RM can be tested, or it can be estimated based on other loads and reps. There are many online resources to estimate your 1 RM and I've found them, for the most part, to be reliable and accurate. If you do a quick google search for "1 RM Calculator," some tools will come up for you to check out.

The 1 RM can also be used to estimate other rep schemes, which online calculators can help determine. For example, if you have a 1 RM of 200 pounds, your 5 RM weight would be approximately 170 pounds or 85%.

INTENSITY

Intensity is expressed as a percentage of your 1 RM. It is the amount of weight used in an exercise.

For a 300 pound max squat, an intensity of 85% would be 255.

Intensities are often used in the purposeful progression and planning of a strength-training program and used to prescribe training loads on given days.

HYPERTROPHY

Hypertrophy is the increase in size of muscle fibers.

Bodybuilders typically demonstrate the most significant increases in muscular hypertrophy.

There are 2 basic types of hypertrophy. Although we cannot exclusively train for one of the other, we can preferentially train for one over the other with approaches outlined in this book.

The difference basically comes down to structure vs. function in how we approach training.

MYOFIBRILLAR HYPERTROPHY

This is structural enlargement of muscle fibers (myofibrills) when the fibers become higher quality and are able to generate more force. This leads to a higher quality, dense muscle tissue.

SARCOPLASMIC HYPERTROPHY

This is an increase in volume of the fluid (the sarcoplasm) in the muscle cell with no concurrent increase in strength gains.

Again, we can't "exclusively" train for one type over the other, a more functional training approach, like *The Edge of Strength*, helps to build more myofibrillar hypertrophy.

Think of myofibrillar hypertrophy as the high-quality, functionally strong muscle we want, whereas sarcoplasmic hypertrophy is the "all show and no go" muscle.

We know that larger muscles produce more force and thereby are stronger. But, at the cellular level, myofibrillar hypertrophy is a better quality muscle tissue that is able to produce more force.

PROGRESSIVE OVERLOAD

Progressive overload is the gradual increase of stress placed upon the body during exercise training. We'll discuss this further in the next chapter as it is very important for strength gain and for size.

This is how we make progress. But, we also must understand that we cannot keep stressing the body to no end. This is where proper programming comes into play, which we'll discuss later as well.

Progressive overload can include the manipulation of many variables that can be used for progression, such as:

- **intensity**
- **volume**
- **frequency**
- **duration**

Progressive overload is key, but it has to be used intelligently and cannot be used indefinitely.

DE-LOAD

After a period of structured training that incorporates progressive overload, the de-load is critical as a way to strategically back off of training.

A de-load is a brief period of lower-intensity training that follows a specific training cycle or program (a periodized approach).

This is what makes the principle of progressive overload successful, and as I just mentioned, we cannot train continuously using progressive overload. In other words, **we can't go all out, all the time.**

Proper "de-loading," or recovery, periods are essential and required to make further progress.

PERIODIZATION

In the simplest terms, periodization is planning for the short and long term.

MACROCYCLE: A 1-YEAR TRAINING PLAN

This is the long-term training plan that's mostly implemented by athletes.

Most people typically don't plan their training this far out. It's mostly done for competitive athletes.

But, what if they did?

What if more of us approached our training from a long-term planning perspective?

It could radically improve our focus and outcomes.

MESOCYCLE: TYPICALLY A 2 TO 6 WEEK TRAINING CYCLE

This is the most common approach when someone uses a specific training program for a short time period.

MICROCYCLE: TYPICALLY A 1 WEEK OR LESS TRAINING CYCLE

This is the smallest training period implemented in training cycles.

We'll discuss the importance of periodization and how I use it in Section IV.

EXCESS POST-EXERCISE OXYGEN CONSUMPTION (EPOC)

This is an important concept to understand.

After higher intensity exercise, the amount of oxygen consumed can be elevated for several hours.

The more intense the exercise (as done with heavy weight training), the more the energy and metabolic cost that will persist post-training.

What this means is your metabolism can be elevated for many hours after training.

In comparison to low-intensity exercise (running, for example), oxygen is consumed during the exercise itself, so the metabolic cost is during the exercise, not after the exercise.

The bottom line is that heavy strength training ramps up our metabolism to a far greater extent and for a more prolonged time period than anything else. That's EPOC.

THE 3 ENERGY SYSTEMS

We have 3 energy systems in our body to drive performance, and how this relates to conditioning will be discussed later in the book.

As we discuss training methods and tools, it will be important to understand these 3 energy systems and how they impact our training.

Here's a brief review.

ATP-CR SYSTEM (ANAEROBIC ALACTIC ENERGY SYSTEM)

This energy system is used in the first 10 seconds or so of exercise and ATP is the primary energy source here.

Strength sports, which requires short bursts, rely heavily on this system. Think of the 40-yard dash or an explosive barbell snatch for 1 rep.

GLYCOLYTIC (ANAEROBIC LACTIC ENERGY SYSTEM)

The glycolytic system comes into play AFTER the initial 10 seconds of exercise and lasts up to about 2 minutes of training to meet energy requirements.

Think of 200 to 400 meter runs or a few minutes of kettlebell swings or snatches.

AEROBIC (AEROBIC ENERGY SYSTEM)

Beyond the first 2 minutes of an exercise, energy must then come from the oxidative pathway. Energy is generated in the mitochondria, which is our intracellular powerhouse for all energy production.

Examples here are long runs, low-level long walks, and long-distance swimming.

All 3 energy systems can used, depending on the exercise variables and duration of the exercise.

THE MOTOR UNIT

The motor unit is the basic element of motor system output.

It is the nerve cell (or motor neuron) that extends from the spinal cord (CNS) to all the muscle fibers that it innervates.

Strength training is a neuromuscular process. When the motor unit is recruited, it activates the muscle fibers to contract.

Anyone who trains for strength will greatly benefit from increasing muscle fiber activation; this is the key to strength development.

MUSCLE FIBER TYPES

SLOW-TWITCH MUSCLE FIBERS

Type I Slow Twitch

Slow twitch (or red fibers) are our muscle fibers that are resistant to fatigue but have low force output. These are essentially the muscle fibers that allow for endurance events.

FAST-TWITCH MUSCLE FIBERS

Type IIa Fast Twitch (Intermediate)

Fast twitch (or white fibers) are the muscle fibers that are primarily responsible for fast, explosive, and powerful muscle contractions.

Type IIx Fast Twitch

These fibers are the strongest, but also have almost no resistance to fatigue. The type II muscle fibers are the ones that are most important for strength training.

Muscle fiber type is a deep subject, and it's important to at least know what muscle fiber types we're training and working on with the qualities of strength development.

NEUROMUSCULAR EFFICIENCY

Neuromuscular efficiency (NME) refers to the ability of the nervous system to properly recruit the appropriate muscles to produce and reduce force.

This is the communication and interaction of the nervous system and muscular system to produce movement.

Additionally, it allows us to dynamically stabilize the body in all planes of movement.

As we train and improve our skills, we improve our neuromuscular efficiency, which makes us more skilled athletes with enhanced movement quality.

Consider the impact of the communication between the nervous system and muscular system, and you'll become a better mover through neuromuscular efficiency. This is why we practice.

Improving NME benefits our movement, strength, power, and other skills related to performance.

PERSONAL RECORD (PR)

A personal record or personal best in a lift is the best you've ever performed.

Your current 1 RM and your personal PR can be 2 different things.

There are many ways to hit new PRs such as with new lifts, with additional skills, within a given year or time frame, or even with specific volume or density sessions (volume = sets x weight; density = volume/time).

As a strength athlete or lifter, you're always looking for new PRs in some way in your training.

COMPENSATORY ACCELERATION TECHNIQUE

I'm bringing up this term and technique because I've personally had success with it. For example, this technique helped me hit a new PR in deadlifting.

Compensatory acceleration technique (C.A.T.) is an effective technique to increase strength, but it's something that requires practice and learning to optimize the benefits.

It's done by lifting submaximal loads explosively, thereby improving ability to generate force production.

This is the specific technique that has been popularized and successfully implemented by Dr. Fred Hatfield, who I was honored to interview on **The Rdella Training® Podcast.**

The deadlift is a great example of how to use C.A.T. For example, you'd perform a deadlift with 70% load, and pull as fast and as explosively as possible.

As the load increases, the more you will lose this speed and explosiveness. However, my experience is that there is carryover from these techniques that improves overall strength development.

The quality of explosive strength is extremely important and we'll cover the 9 qualities of strength later (Chapter 4).

A GRIND

A grind is a slower, more controlled movement. Grinds are the slow lifts, such as deadlifts, squats, and presses.

A BALLISTIC

A ballistic is a fast, explosive movement.

Kettlebell ballistics are kettlebell swings, snatches, and cleans.

And in Olympic Weightlifting, they are the barbell clean and jerks and snatches.

GPP AND SPP

It's very important to understand 2 distinct training approaches.

- General Physical Preparation (GGP)
- Special Physical Preparation (SPP)

GPP is training very broadly for general fitness. It's a generalized approach, training to improve many different fitness components and qualities that are applied to a wide range of tasks.

Today, the easiest way to think of GPP is with CrossFit style training, where you do a lot of different things without specializing in any specific area. It's a broad-based training approach.

SPP is a specialized way to train. It applies the law of specificity, which means we train a specific way for a specific goal.

"If everything is a priority, then nothing is a priority," according to Coach Rob Lawrence.

The point is if you want to great at anything, you do have to prioritize or specialize.

That's exactly the approach I've used with great success as you'll see in Strength Stacking in Section IV.

Both GPP and SPP have important roles, of course.

It's important to note there is overlap between GPP and SPP, and only elite athletes will truly specialize with an SPP approach as competition approaches.

For example, Olympic weightlifting can have both GPP and SPP components if using the lifts in a generalized fitness training approach.

If using Olympic lifts to prepare for competition, then you are preparing with an SPP approach.

True examples of SPP could include:

- Competitive Olympic weightlifting
- Girevoy Sport (Kettlebells)
- Competitive powerlifting (or single-event powerlifting)

Do you take a GPP approach or SPP approach?

GPP and SPP both serve purposes, which one you use should depend on your goals and can change depending on training priorities.

This chapter provided some important terms and concepts to consider in moving forward in the book.

In the next chapter, we're going to answer one of the most important questions in strength training that gets little attention.

CHAPTER 4: HOW STRONG IS STRONG ENOUGH?

"You can be strong or you can be weak."
–Louie Simmons

Look around, my friend. If you're strong, you're in the minority.

But, how strong do you need to become?

What qualifies as **strong enough** is the burning question I've been obsessed with answering.

But when we talk about strength, we should be asking what type of strength we are referring to.

It's important to understand that there are many different qualities of strength.

Each quality will be dependent on the athlete or individual's training goal.

Understanding the different aspects of strength will help you understand how important it is to be stronger – whether for athletics, recreational activities or to improve quality of life.

First, we'll look at the 9 qualities of strength, then look to answer the question of how strong is strong enough.

9 QUALITIES OF STRENGTH

Strength is the ability to generate force, but there are several types you should understand to better know what type of strength is most important for you and your goals.

There are essentially 9 different types of strength according to the classic book *Supertraining* by Yuri Verkhoshansky and Mel Siff.

ABSOLUTE STRENGTH

First, absolute strength and maximum strength are often used synonymously, however, they are different things according to Dr. Vladimar Zatsiorsky in the great book *The Science and Practice of Strength Training* which I highly recommend.

This gets confusing, so let's try to sort it out.

Absolute strength is the greatest muscular force that can be involuntarily generated. Involuntarily is the key word here.

You might be wondering how this is possible.

Maximum involuntary muscular contraction can be achieved under the influence of electrical stimulation (ES) or stimulated by other means.

So, absolute strength is maximum involuntary contraction.

Honestly, absolute strength is almost a meaningless term.

How could you achieve it since none of us will be undergoing training under electrical stimulation?

The more accurate term is maximum strength.

MAXIMUM STRENGTH (OR LIMIT STRENGTH)

Again, maximum strength and absolute strength are very often referred to as being the same when they are not, at least if we go by the definition by Dr. Zatsiorsky and others.

You know how people ask, "how much can you bench?" As ridiculous as that question is, it's asking the question of maximum strength.

Maximum strength is the muscle force that can be voluntarily produced.

More specifically, it's the maximum muscular force that can be produced without a time limit or a limit to the amount of weight lifted.

A current 500-pound maximum deadlift is an example of maximum strength, regardless of bodyweight.

How much weight can you maximally lift in a given exercise on your best day? That's maximum strength.

If you're a powerlifter, you are a specialist in the development of maximal strength.

RELATIVE STRENGTH

This is strength as it relates to a person's bodyweight (BW).

A deadlift of 3 times bodyweight is an example of relative strength.

And, relative strength is an excellent indicator of how strong an individual really is.

For example, a 500-pound deadlift is much more impressive for an athlete who weighs 160 pounds (>3x BW) as compared to the athlete who weighs 250 (2x BW) – something to keep in mind.

A 600-pound deadlift is extremely impressive, without a doubt. But, if you have an athlete who weighs 300 pounds and another who weighs 160 pounds and they both pull 600, who's DL is more impressive?

That's relative strength.

EXPLOSIVE STRENGTH

Explosive strength is the ability to produce maximal force in minimal time. It's producing maximal force as quickly as possible.

Explosive strength is most characteristically involved in athletics.

Almost all athletes need this type of strength to be successful.

Yet it's NOT only for athletes, but useful for all of us. I'll tell you why later in the book.

Examples are Olympic weightlifting, the kettlebell ballistic exercises, and certain bodyweight exercises, just to name a few.

STRENGTH ENDURANCE

Strength endurance is the ability to sustain qualities of strength for an extended period of time.

This is one of the most important qualities of strength – if not the most important for some of us.

It's the ability to be able to sustain muscle function for a long duration.

Depending on who you read, it has also been termed "work capacity" because it allows work to be done for sustained time periods.

Strength endurance is conditioning. Conditioning is very important, especially for combat athletes and many other types of athletes.

Digging deeper into this quality, it's important to note that there are 2 different types of strength endurance.

STATIC STRENGTH ENDURANCE:

Static strength-endurance implies isometric tension of varying magnitude and duration, or in holding a certain posture.

Static strength endurance is associated with relatively long or short term sustained muscular tension, and it's duration in each case is determined by its magnitude.

Think of the plank exercise or pause squats where no movement is being done, but isometric muscle contraction is being held for an extended period of time.

DYNAMIC STRENGTH ENDURANCE:

Dynamic strength endurance is typically associated with cyclic exercises in which considerable tension is repeated without interruption during each cycle of movement.

Think of cycling, rowing, or performing a 5-minute kettlebell snatch test.

It is also present in acyclic events requiring maximum power repetitions with short rest periods between, such as jumping or throwing activities.

STARTING STRENGTH

Starting strength is the ability of the muscles to generate force at the beginning of a lift.

The deadlift is a great example of when you need starting strength to generate force **off of the floor.**

Isometric muscle action occurs first to initiate the movement.

SPEED-STRENGTH

Speed-strength is generally reserved for athletic events or activities in which power is generated with body mass or light loads.

Speed strength training is typically done with no resistance or very light external resistance.

These techniques were developed by Russian sports scientists to enhance the development of power for athletes.

A great example would be a sprinter who becomes stronger to specifically increase sprint performance; they would demonstrate the quality of speed-strength.

STRENGTH-SPEED

Strength-speed is a training technique to move heavier loads faster.

It's generating power against heavier loads.

This can also be considered dynamic effort training to generate more speed with sub-maximal loads.

An example is sub-maximal deadlifts (~60-70% 1 RM) that are lifted faster or explosively.

This training technique has been used for some time to develop rate of force development and explosive strength.

ACCELERATION STRENGTH

Acceleration strength is different from explosive strength.

Acceleration strength is the ability to quickly increase force <u>at the beginning</u> of the movement.

THE 5 LEVELS OF STRENGTH

How strong is strong enough?

Can someone have too much strength?

I believe the 5 levels of strength answer these major questions.

L1: UN-STRENGTH

L2: THRESHOLD STRENGTH

L3: FOUNDATIONAL STRENGTH

L4: AGGRESSIVE STRENGTH

L5: SUPER STRENGTH

THE 5 LEVELS OF STRENGTH

None of us want to have Level 1 strength, and very few of us will be at Level 5 strength.

You'll fully understand what I mean after reading this section and hopefully you'll be clear on where you need to be for your specific training goals.

LEVEL 1: UN-STRENGTH

This is the level when a person doesn't have enough strength to operate at a normal level.

Level 1 includes the ill-health or severely de-conditioned individual.

Imagine an elderly person who has lost their strength and is no longer able to function independently.

The person who has trouble getting up and out of a chair and walking.

This may not always be the elderly, though.

For example, when you get sick with the flu, what happens?

You lose your strength fast. You may go the level of un-strength. That's what has happened to me when I've felt so bad it's hard to get up and even walk to the kitchen.

This is when you quickly realize how important strength really is just to function on a day-to-day level. When you lose the ability to function normally, it's frightening.

Unfortunately, I've seen many younger and middle-aged people who are extremely de-conditioned due to lack of exercise and poor diet. It's painful to witness let alone to live.

Yes, it is inevitable for us to lose strength as we age, but we can prevent or significantly slow the process be engaging is regular strength training for as long as we can.

Un-strength is lack of strength that inhibits function.

However, unless you are suffering a health condition that limits your function and zaps all your energy, you can get from here to the next level.

LEVEL 2: THRESHOLD STRENGTH

Threshold strength is the strength we need to function normally on a day-to-day basis. This is where most people are who don't exercise at all.

People who do not engage in regular strength training, but are not limited functionally are Level 2.

This means that they can go about their typical day to walk around and move.

They have threshold strength to function, whereas un-strength does not even account for that.

This level does not require any strength training at all. Think about how many people you know who don't exercise, but they are functioning just fine.

They live their life, they have no significant issues with errands, and they are operating on a baseline of strength that provides them enough to function day in and day out.

But, they are not optimizing their performance or potential. This lack of strength development will be detrimental to health and life, not to mention it's dangerously close to Level 1.

LEVEL 3: FOUNDATIONAL STRENGTH

Foundational strength is the minimum level everyone should strive for.

This level is general strength training or GPP (general physical preparation).

Some people may have no desire to move beyond this level, but this is the minimum or baseline level for a lifetime of optimal health and performance.

This level is "foundational" and has no age limits or restrictions.

The majority of people who engage in regular exercise training are found at this level. It's the basic strength we get from working out on a consistent basis.

This is the strength we gain above threshold strength, as opposed to not exercising at all, where strength loss is on a progressive decline.

The person here may just workout because they want to get "fit," to look better, and to feel better.

Nobody at Level 3 is training to be superhuman, but they know they need some form of strength training in their health and fitness equation.

In other words, they get stronger because it's part of their program, but not in an overly aggressive way.

Here are some examples of those that are found in this level:

- Recreational exercisers
- Endurance athletes who incorporate strength training
- Certain athletes, not needing high levels of strength
- Generalists (does different things to be "generally" fit)
- Most fat-loss programming
- Non-competitive CrossFitters
- "Bootcampers"
- Bodybuilders (depending on program or phase)
- Many broad-based strength and conditioning programs

You might be wondering about some of the examples above, but you'll see the difference in the next level.

What does this look like from a training standpoint?

People at this level may do the standard 3 sets of 10 of an exercise with "moderate" weight.

Often they intentionally do not train heavy for fear of bulking or becoming excessively strong (false beliefs).

They go to the gym a few times a week, they engage in strength training, and they feel better as a result.

Preventing weakness and de-conditioning are major benefits of this level of foundational strength.

It's the generalized and broad approach to strength for most of us.

But, getting seriously strong isn't part of this level. Heavy training won't be part of a Level 3 training routine.

This involves either maintaining or developing general strength; this level is definitely not losing it.

Foundational strength is a baseline and lays the groundwork for health, for aesthetics, and for performance.

But, it's not to be confused with Level 4.

LEVEL 4: AGGRESSIVE STRENGTH

This is where the individual takes strength training much more seriously. This is training stronger than the "average Joe".

The level of specialization in strength becomes more dominant.

No longer are people generalists because they begin to focus more on the strength qualities and to become physically stronger for specific goals.

This is the "next level" of strength and performance.

Strength goals are more objective and specific.

In simple terms, **people here are training more aggressively for the purpose of getting stronger.**

They want to be stronger, and they better understand the value of strength qualities.

Today, I believe there are more fitness enthusiasts moving towards this level, as people understand the importance of getting stronger (and if you're reading this, you're one of them).

Aggressive strength may involve training with barbells, heavy kettlebells, advanced bodyweight and gymnastics type movements, and even "hardcore" bodybuilding types of programming.

Maximum strength, explosive strength, and strength endurance are some examples of strength qualities being purposefully developed at this level.

Athletes here are working on power, speed, and skill development. Examples could be:

- Contact sports athletes
- Competitive CrossFit athletes

- People with specific strength goals
- "Off Season" weightlifting and powerlifting
- Certain bodybuilding programs
- Training for advanced fitness certifications (SFG/SFL/RKC for example)
- Track and field athletes (*season dependent)
- Other athletes requiring higher levels of strength and power

What does this look like?

It's training with rep schemes of 3-5 reps with heavy loads, focusing on the skill of strength.

Skills are developed, performance increases, and more specific programming progressions evolve.

People at this level are pushing and testing their limits.

Consistency, hard training, program planning, periodization, and progressive overload are some of the principles involved at this level.

The athlete may be training for an athletic event, higher level certification, or simply to attain a specific objective goal or set of goals.

There is a **greater drive, desire,** and **motivation** at this level to become stronger beyond foundational strength.

LEVEL 5: SUPER STRENGTH

This is the elite level.

This is where the individual intentionally seeks maximum performance and the highest levels of strength.

Remember, there are many different qualities of strength.

Some qualities of strength include:

- Limit or maximum strength
- Strength endurance
- Explosive strength

Professional strength athletes, amateur strength athletes, and anyone competing in strength or power events will likely be at this level.

They are training and peaking specifically to reach their strength performance potential.

You don't necessarily have to be a competitor to be at this level. However, most will seek to achieve the level of super strength because they either want to compete or want to accomplish a clearly defined objective or performance goal.

Super strength is training at a very high level to move as close as possible toward the individual's strength level potential.

It's training exclusively to be as strong (or explosive) as you can. Examples include:

- Explosive strength (Competitive Olympic weightlifting)
- Maximum strength (Powerlifting or strong man)
- Strength endurance (Kettlebell sport)
- Speed, acceleration, explosiveness (Football)
- Speed strength, power, explosiveness (Track and field athletes, season dependent)
- Other strength/power-specific sports and athletics

Again, this is the highest level of specialized strength training to achieve specific performance abilities.

This is competition level.

This is elite level.

This is rare and exclusive.

REVIEW OF THE 5 LEVELS

We all fall into 1 of these 5 levels. So how strong is strong enough?

If you engage in consistent strength training, you should be able to answer this question.

How strong do you need to be for the goals you want?

It's important to understand where you are now and what you can achieve.

Because my goals are to help more people get more specific results, it's important to understand these levels of strength and know how strong is strong enough for YOU.

Personally, I lived with foundational strength for many years. But, I also stayed in a "plateau" until I better understood the value of taking my strength and performance to a higher level.

Anyone can greatly benefit from Level 3 – Foundational Strength.

As you and I experience our own personal journey, we should be able to answer the important question, how strong is strong enough – for the specific goals we want.

It's simple and useful to understand these 5 levels.

What level is most appropriate for you right now?

It goes back to being clear on your primary training purpose.

It is very likely for you to transition up or down between the levels, depending on the current goals and training cycles.

For example, when I competed in powerlifting, I went from a level 4 to a level 5, based on a shift in my training goals.

Training goals will tell you where you should be.

How strong is strong enough?

It all depends on where your goals fit into 1 of the 5 levels of strength.

Understanding this simple concept will help with short-term and long-term planning and how you approach your training.

STRENGTH STANDARDS

Now that you understand the 5 levels of strength, it's also important to understand some basic "standards."

Standards are basic strength or performance "levels" that should be met.

Standards should be based on age, gender, training background, and other factors.

Take them for what they are.

There are many standards out there.

Of course, it would be inappropriate to suggest that all humans should be able to deadlift 500 pounds.

That's not a realistic or advisable strength for most of us, is it?

While that would be awesome and amazing for many people, it would be unfair to suggest that as a standard for everyone, regardless of age or training experience.

Here's some outstanding examples of what's "strong enough" from various strength coaches:

MIKE BOYLE STRENGTH STANDARDS.

Bench press: 1.25 to 1.5 x bodyweight (250 to 300 pounds for a 200-pound athlete)

Clean: 1.25 to 1.5 x bodyweight (same as above)

Front squat: 1.5 to 1.75 x bodyweight (300 to 350 pounds for a 200-pound athlete)

MARK RIPPETOE'S BARBELL STANDARDS.

http://startingstrength.com/files/standards.pdf

GREG EVERETT OF CATALYST ATHLETICS.

http://www.catalystathletics.com/article/1836/Olympic-Weightlifting-Skill-Levels-Chart/

DAN JOHN'S STANDARDS.

MEN (THESE ARE HIS "GAME CHANGER" STANDARDS)

- Bodyweight bench press for 15 reps
- 15 pull-ups
- Bodyweight squat for 15 reps
- Double bodyweight deadlift
- Farmer's walks with "bodyweight" per hand

WOMEN (THESE ARE HIS "GAME CHANGER" STANDARDS)

- Bodyweight bench press
- 3 pull-ups
- 275-pound deadlift
- 135 pound squat for 5 reps
- Farmer's walks with 85 pounds per hand

Depending on what your training goals are, these may be very helpful for understanding strength standards and where you should be.

If you do some research, you'll find more standards specific to age, gender, and fitness task.

One last time, how strong is strong enough?

It all depends, but this chapter has provided some guidance and considerations to be able to answer that important question.

Next, we'll explore why we all need to work on hypertrophy to achieve our individual goals.

I'll explain why we all need more muscle.

CHAPTER 5: WE ALL NEED MUSCLE MASS

"Hypertrophy and joint mobility trump everything else."
–Dan John

Do you know about the culprit of aging called sarcopenia?

Most people begin to lose modest amounts of muscle mass after the age of 30 with resultant loss of strength.

This progressive loss of skeletal muscle that comes with aging is called **sarcopenia.**

Muscle wasting is devastating, and it's shocking that we don't hear more about it.

We all age, right? Well, that means we're all susceptible to sarcopenia. And the research about it is frightening.

I'll tell you why you should be scared as hell about losing muscle mass and why putting on muscle is much harder than you can imagine.

Yet, there exists this fear of bulking, which is a false fear. It's hard to pack on mass.

For some reason, people are misinformed about strength training and think that if they train heavy or hard, they will excessively bulk up.

This is the **fear of bulking.** But what you should have is the fear of sarcopenia.

The truth is that building enough muscle to bulk requires consuming a ton of food and training a very specific way.

Bulking up is extremely difficult.

The fact is we all need to work on muscle building, aka hypertrophy. This is an increase in size of skeletal muscle through a growth in size of its component cells.

A major part my goal with this book is to provide a long-term training approach for lifetime success, not just getting results in the near future.

It doesn't matter how young or how old you are, you need to understand the lifetime benefits of strength training, specifically as it relates to muscle tissue.

There's a lot more to strength than just "getting stronger."

Strength training may be the single most potent way to combat the effects of aging, and if there's a fountain of youth, this is it.

What else can significantly improve our health, function, and youthful presence to the extent of a properly designed strength training program?

LOSS OF PHYSICAL POWER

The loss of physical power is a big deal.

First of all, it just sounds scary. I mean, who would want to consciously lose their physical power?

Nobody.

Power production is an important physical attribute that we need, even as we get older.

Athletes especially need power or the ability to generate force quickly. But we need this as we age because power also relates to functional activities.

Do you want to get up slowly out of a chair and struggle, or would you prefer to bounce up from the chair with vibrancy, energy, and even power?

The ability to generate force quickly will always be a desirable and necessary attribute.

There is a need to continue to develop the quality of power over a lifetime to optimize functional performance.

It helps us to perform better not only in athletics but in daily life.

SARCOPENIA (MUSCLE WASTING)

Sarcopenia is the loss of muscle fiber size and mass that results in a loss of strength as we age.

Yes, it is part of the normal aging process, but **we can blunt the effects of sarcopenia with strength and power training.**

Here's what happens to our muscle tissue from a cellular level. As most people age and become more inactive or sedentary, this propagates apoptosis.

Apoptosis is programmed cell death.

This means our muscle cells die with inactivity which leads to increased sarcopenia.

Inactivity enhances sarcopenia, which leads to loss of muscle function and greater risk for major health issues, functional decline, and a higher rate of morality.

It's a vicious cycle.

Loss of muscle mass is related to metabolic conditions such as insulin resistance and Type II Diabetes.

And, reducing the incidence of sarcopenia could save the population millions of dollars in healthcare costs.

The direct cause of sarcopenia is unclear.

Although sarcopenia is <u>mostly</u> seen in people who are inactive, it can occur in people who stay physically active.

This suggests there are other factors involved in the development of sarcopenia.

Reported factors include:

- Loss of alpha motor neurons
- Decrease in muscle cell contractility
- Decrease in the concentrations of hormones such as growth hormone (GH), testosterone (T) and insulin-like growth factor (IGF1)
- Decrease in the body's ability to synthesize protein
- Inadequate intake of calories and/or protein to sustain muscle mass
- Increases in production of catabolic agents (cytokines)

Where does this leave us as we get older? How can fight off the devastating effects of sarcopenia?

We get stronger with the right exercise.

We protect our bodies through strategic and fundamental strength training.

Strength and power training, as presented in *The Edge of Strength*, can greatly influence the function and integrity of the underlying cells, muscle, other connective tissues, and physiological systems.

By positively influencing these structures and systems, we will maximize our potential to maintain a high level of function and performance for a stronger life.

FIBER TYPES AND HYPERTROPHY

Studies have suggested that strength loss is mainly attributed to a decrease in muscle mass.

Indeed, we all need hypertrophy.

The more muscle we lose, the more force production we lose.

Specifically, **we tend to lose more of the type II (fast twitch) muscle fibers**, which are the fibers responsible for our explosive strength and power. This is NOT what we want to lose.

If we stop training, there appears to be a **selective atrophy of the type II muscle fiber.**

Most people do not realize the importance of preserving the quality of explosive strength, but this is critically important for health, function, and performance.

We want to exhibit power for as long as we can. The only way to minimize this loss and decrease in the type II muscle fiber is through a lifetime of strength training, specifically using the methods covered in Section IV.

To understand why it all works, though, I'll cover the powerful science to support this in the next chapter.

No matter what your age, it's crucial to understand the physiological consequences of not being strong because it can literally kill us.

If you have any fear of bulking, please let it go.

We need muscle.

We need muscle to protect our bodies, preserve our strength, and maximize our health.

CHAPTER 6: STRENGTH SCIENCE

"Tough times don't last. Tough people do."
-Bruce Arians

Today, longevity is becoming much more talked about in the health and fitness industry.

The average life expectancy in the U.S. is 78 years old. Can we actually live longer than that by becoming stronger?

No one can say for sure, but it seems to make sense. And there's even science behind it.

I remember being in a conversation with a well-known strength expert. It was an amazing discussion, and he made a comment about the relationship between strength and longevity.

What he was talking about was maximum strength.

There is very strong evidence that being stronger will, in fact, help us to live longer, healthier, and more vibrant lives.

This doesn't mean we all need to have 500-pound deadlifts to live longer.

But, we need to have and maintain baseline strength – Level 3 Strength – for as long as possible.

The strongest shall survive the longest, and science demonstrates this. It's scary when you think about the consequences of lack of strength.

SCARY STRENGTH SCIENCE

There is never any guarantee that any one of us will not be stricken with a life-threatening disease.

Nobody is immune to that.

What strength training and good nutrition do is MINIMIZE the risk of any major life-threatening disease.

Does it guarantee it? No.

Does it help prevent it? Yes.

Developing strength helps with healing and recovery when we are ill. It helps us to bounce back faster and battle through adversity.

I recently heard a renowned physician, a longevity expert, say something really profound in an interview.

*"I do think the most important form of exercise is
high-intensity heavy strength training."*

He attributed most of our health problems to our inability to be strong. He's right.

He said we are "de-conditioned" so badly at the muscular level that it greatly impairs our health and function.

He also asked the question: What's the difference between LeBron James today and LeBron in 10 years from now?

The difference is his level of strength. In 10 years he will likely not be as physically strong as he is today. Yes, even LeBron James will be affected by sarcopenia as he ages.

There are benefits of strength that greatly contribute to overall metabolic health. **Strength is a physiological and neuromuscular process which greatly contributes to human health and performance.**

Did you get that?

Strength supports human health as well as performance.

One of the most powerful reasons to be stronger was cited in a landmark study on the association between strength and mortality (i.e., the rate of death) in men.

While the study was an observational study and we can't make absolute conclusions based on the correlation of the findings, the data is certainly convincing and supports what common sense would tell us.

Common sense tells us that **stronger people live longer.**

In a study with nearly 9,000 men, ages 20 to 80, the authors found that muscular strength was significantly and inversely related to risk for death from all causes.

The study also suggested that if you were in the top 3rd in terms of physical strength, you were less likely to die from all causes including disease, accident, or something else.

In other words, the more strength, the lower the chance for risk from death.

This is compelling, but it shouldn't be surprising.

Strength training seems to offer a protective benefit to the risk of death for all causes. It makes the statement "the strongest shall survive" ring true.

If you have a physically strong person and a physically weak person, who is going to be better equipped to deal with the adversity, the challenges, and the punches that life throws at us on almost a daily basis?

The question I always ask is when would being stronger ever be a bad thing?

Who would not benefit by becoming stronger?

You can never really be too strong.

I can't think of a single person, athlete or other, who has ever become "too strong" (although there may be a few individuals out there that I'm not aware of).

But, I can think of MANY who became too weak or de-conditioned and suffered as a result.

Strength would be a hindrance only if it detracted from other important physical qualities such a movement, health, mobility, or athletic performance.

But, remember what we said about the stronger athlete being the better athlete if all things are equal?

Strength training gives us more qualities and makes us better in almost every way.

It's amazing that this simple principle is often completely missed or misunderstood. The stronger person will overcome more than the weaker person.

Here's something else that's really interesting about strength and muscle.

Did you know that approximately 30% of skeletal muscle mass is lost between the 5th and 8th decades of life?

A THIRD OF SKELETAL MUSCLE IS LOST AFTER YOUR 40'S.

That is serious, my fellow fitness enthusiast.

That loss in muscle tissue is significant, and this is the reason we need to work on hypertrophy (muscle building) as we get older.

I guess you could say that we all need to become bodybuilders, at least at some level.

Tell me again that you don't want to add too much muscle.

Muscle protects us in more ways that we can imagine.

It not only makes us stronger but keeps us healthier to function at a high level in all aspects of our lives.

Why does this massive loss of muscle mass occur?

This reduction as we age happens for several reasons:

- Sedentary lifestyle (or decreased activity)
- Malnutrition
- Insulin resistance (insulin fails to function normally, thereby becomes resistant)
- Oxidative stress (damage at the cellular level)
- Alterations in skeletal muscle metabolism and repair

We need to do everything we can by way of movement, exercise, nutrition, supplementation, stress management, and more to minimize this from happening.

This isn't rocket science, folks, but it is science.

We all know the importance of exercise and nutrition. Unfortunately, the majority of people fail to implement the simple things, the fundamental principles for optimal health and fitness.

One last study I'll point out was another groundbreaker about the importance of strength.

A more recent study in 2011 evaluated muscular strength and all-cause mortality in 1506 hypertensive men who were 40 years old or older.

The findings were similar to the previous study in that higher levels of muscular strength correlated to lower risk of death for all causes through 18 years of follow-up.

Strength seems to be protective, according to these studies.

THE SCIENCE OF GETTING STRONGER

Now, we'll look at how we get stronger using science.

The science of strength development is important to understand because when you understand how it works, strength becomes easier to develop.

You already know that **bigger muscles are able to produce more force.** Typically, the bigger the muscle, the stronger the muscle, so size does matter.

But, we also need the right type of training to produce denser, higher quality muscle tissue – that's myofibrillar hypertrophy.

Strength is really a process of the nervous system.

To get stronger, we should understand the basic neural mechanisms. The explanation is a little scientific, but it's important to understand.

The simple explanation is that we recruit more muscle fibers through deliberate practice.

We have to practice the skill of strength.

The central nervous system (CNS) is a fascinating and critical component in the process of strength development.

The CNS consists of the brain and spinal cord, while the peripheral nervous system (PNS) is all the other nerves in our body.

We get stronger by increasing the firing potential of our motor neurons and motor units.

A **motor neuron** is essentially a nerve cell that connects or innervates a muscle.

A single motor neuron may innervate many muscle fibers. There's a cellular mechanism (called an action potential) that occurs to activate the muscle which makes the muscle contract.

The motor neuron and all the muscle fibers that are innervated are called the **motor unit.**

The more we can influence the firing of the motor unit, the stronger we get.

The real question is, how do we do that? Luckily the answer is simple.

First, we train with heavier loads.

To get stronger, we train stronger and regularly practice the skill of strength. We need to lift heavy weights to stimulate and activate the motor neuron.

The key is to optimally recruit the motor unit firing.

Here's how that works.

Strong athletes appropriately activate their muscular systems to increase the firing patterns through neural adaptation.

Neural adaptation is maximally recruiting or activating the nervous system. This is learned and developed with practicing proper techniques under heavier loads.

Olympic weightlifting is a perfect example of neural adaptation.

Since increases in strength are due to neural adaptation, strength truly is a skill, and it's one that can be trained and developed by anyone with proper training.

Yes, strength can be attained by anyone who desires to become stronger.

I'll say it again: **strength can be attained by anyone who desires to become stronger.**

This is really important to understand because strength can be acquired through practice, just like any other skill.

After reading this book, who wouldn't want to get stronger?

The more we "practice" our techniques and skills, the stronger we will become, it's that simple.

Practicing the skill of strength will get you stronger by increasing the potential of the neuromuscular system.

Specifically, the more we can recruit our muscular system with simple techniques such as increasing muscular tension, we will increase our motor unit activation.

These techniques will build strength over time by neural adaptation (increasing the efficiency of our nervous system).

We can literally program our bodies to get stronger.

Strength training can be considered a neuromuscular process to enhance our gross motor activities.

This means strength training allows us to move better and perform better because of the effect and interaction of the nervous system and muscular system, which influences performance.

Basically, we are conditioning both our nervous system and muscular system for strength development over time.

Applying the concept of neural adaptation is how we get stronger.

We must generate large numbers of motor unit activation and have them fire at an optimal level.

Then, we can produce an output that approaches our **strength potential.**

Another important point is that with increased force and power production, the **firing rate** of the motor units are increased.

What this means is not only do the number of motor units increase but the rate at which they fire increases, which also contributes to maximal force production.

There is also evidence that if the motor units fire in **synchronization** (in a certain order), this may contribute to maximal strength development as well.

The bottom line is that strength is a result of conditioning our central nervous system (CNS) to develop the improved firing and communication between our muscular system.

So then, strength is the effective **communication** and **activation** between our nervous system and our muscular system.

How do you use and apply this information?

The practical application is simply to recognize that strength is a skill that needs to be developed and improved by deliberate practice.

Let's talk about practice.

DELIBERATE PRACTICE AND MYELIN

Myelin is an insulator in our nervous system. It allows nerve impulses or signals to travel faster. What's interesting is that myelin grows in proportion to the hours we spend with practice.

Every time we perform a rep, we potentially build another layer of myelin to our nervous system.

The more we practice, the more myelin our bodies develop.

What does this mean?

The more you practice, the more myelin you produce, and the more you develop your skills.

Myelin growth is linked to improved athletic performance.

This is fascinating, don't you think? For more on the science of myelin, see the work of Daniel Coyle in *The Talent Code.*

Focus on deliberate practice to rebuild your nervous system with myelin growth.

According to the science of strength development, the application and combination of these points will get you stronger:

- Proper technique
- Applying increased muscular tension
- Deliberate practice
- Focusing on generating more muscle fiber recruitment

Once again, strength truly is a skill that can be developed by anyone who wishes to become stronger.

At this point, you now understand more of the WHY we need to be strong and HOW it can be acquired.

SECTION II – APPROACHING STRENGTH

*"You have the personal obligation to yourself
to make yourself the best product possible, according to your own terms.
Not the biggest or most successful, but the best quality – with that
achieved, comes everything else."*
–Bruce Lee

CHAPTER 7: MOVE WELL

"The body is designed to work wholly and interactively and function as a system – different muscle groups working together in a coordinated fashion, rather than separately in stunted, isolated motion."
–Dave Draper

Before we move strong, we must move well.

How can we improve movement before getting stronger?

We need to strive for high-quality movement, not only in training but in our day-to-day activity.

Focus first on being supple, mobile, stable, and agile.

Move well and then move often, as renowned physical therapist Gray Cook states.

In this chapter, we'll review basic principles and assessments of human movement. I'd like to discuss how we can move better and move gracefully.

And, if you already do move well, you need to do everything you can to maintain that suppleness.

In other words, stay on a continuous improvement program for better, optimal movement.

What is good movement?

It should look fluid, effortless, and safe.

High-quality movement means moving with ease through a full range of motion that demonstrates a high degree of mobility, stability, and motor control.

There are many tools and ways we can evaluate and improve human movement.

Let's start at the beginning.

BREATHING

There's a lot of discussion going on about the importance of breathing these days.

That's because any good discussion about optimal movement must begin with the breath.

Breathing is fundamental for human movement, and breathing is fundamental for a high level of athletic performance.

If you carefully evaluate a high-performing and highly successful athlete, you'll notice that their breathing will be effortless, calm, controlled, and efficient.

This is not a coincidence.

It's a significant factor in how that athlete performs in their sport.

Every successful athlete, weightlifter, sprinter, powerlifter, or other strong person will be a master of their breath.

Optimal breathing is effectively using your diaphragm to breathe efficiently, or diaphragmatic breathing.

DIAPHRAGMATIC BREATHING

It's known as belly-breathing as opposed to chest-breathing.

What this looks like is breathing to move the stomach as opposed to breathing from the chest, neck, and upper thorax.

If we're breathing through our chest, we're breathing in a distressed state. It's inefficient, meaning we're doing more work to move oxygen.

Diaphragmatic breathing (or lower abdominal breathing) is easily assessed with this simple exercise.

In a seated or supine position (best in supine), place your hands on the sides of your stomach, and inhale deeply through your nose. You can do this right now.

You should feel your hands move out to the side and to the front as you inhale. In other words, your stomach expands (not your chest) as your breath is inhaled. You will feel your hands sink in as you exhale the air out.

This is diaphragmatic breathing. The diaphragm muscle is functioning optimally in this manner to pull air into the lungs. When the diaphragm relaxes, the air is expelled.

Train yourself to notice what if feels like to diaphragmatically breathe.

We do this by repeated practice and by simply noticing what optimal diaphragmatic breathing is.

Again, this is the way we should be breathing as this is the efficient way to breathe to maximize movement, health, and performance.

It will always be important to assess how you breathe in a relaxed state as well as during exercise and performance.

Again, breathing is the first step in optimal human movement.

BASIC ASSESSMENT OF MOVEMENT

Here are some basic assessment considerations and basic movement patterns to begin with. I recommend getting assessed by a qualified coach, trainer, or movement expert – even if you're a coach or trainer yourself.

Some of what I mention here you can do yourself, but I'd definitely recommend qualified assessment or movement screening.

OBSERVATION

Simply observing how a person moves can tell you a lot.

If you want to know how well you move when you train, take a video of yourself doing a squat, deadlift, press, or any functional movement.

You might be surprised at what you see.

Observation is a skill and something that can be learned.

As a physical therapist, this is something I've been trained in, but you don't have to be trained to notice a **rounded back deadlift** or **poor hip and knee movement** in a squat.

Poor form is often obvious when you pay attention to the details.

There are many things to look at such as posture, movement quality, technical faults, breathing patterns, mobility, and stability.

Again, you do need to know what to look for, but you'd also be surprised about what you might find just by observation.

Anyone can observe what they see.

What do you notice about the way you sit, stand, walk, and carry yourself?

What do you notice about the way you move when you train?

You may be not "trained" to assess posture, but you certainly can make general observations:

Is my head forward, or is my neck tall and aligned?

Are my shoulders rounded forward, or are the shoulder blades pinched back and retracted?

Is my low back slouched, or is there a nice small curve to the low back?

Is my pelvis rotated forward or backward excessively in one way, or am I sitting tall in alignment?

How do I walk? Do I use my arms, are they stiff and rigid or are they relaxed?

THE OVERHEAD SQUAT

The overhead squat is an important assessment tool and part of the functional movement screen, which I'll discuss in just a minute.

But, I like to use the overhead squat (OS) as a stand-alone assessment tool, as well.

The way I like to use the OS is to assess quality of movement: ankle positions, knee positions, spine positions, etc.

While holding a dowel rod (or stick) overhead with hands placed wider than the shoulders, I'll have someone simply perform a full, deep squat while holding the rod or stick overhead.

To perform an overhead squat with full range of motion, an individual needs:

- Sufficient ankle mobility
- Sufficient knee mobility
- Sufficient hip mobility
- Good cervical, thoracic, and lumbar mobility and stability
- Good bilateral shoulder range of motion
- Full elbow extension
- Ability to demonstrate good motor control

This is why it's a good assessment tool as a stand-alone. There's plenty to observe in the overhead squat.

THE FUNCTIONAL MOVEMENT SCREEN

"You can't put fitness on dysfunction."
–Gray Cook

The functional movement screen (FMS) is an extremely valuable tool.

It's a screen, NOT an assessment.

It's a starting point to look for movement deficiencies, but it's not meant to diagnose them.

We need a standardized, reproducible, and repeatable tool to quantify movement and determine if there is a quality movement baseline for safety.

As Gray Cook, the co-creator of the FMS has stated, we screen for health with a blood pressure cuff; yet we don't screen for human movement.

The FMS is that screen.

It's one of the most useful and valuable ways to look at **baseline human movement** and is designed to identify potential risk for injury.

The FMS is 7 basic movement patterns that provide an objective score to screen for red flags, as I see it.

I like to think of the FMS as a **red flag indicator,** meaning that if there are poor movement patterns, we can identify them and work to fix those issues with corrective exercises.

Corrective exercises are simply exercises that are built into a program, specific to the individual in an attempt to correct potential issues.

The FMS is scored on a scale of 0 to 3 in the following:

- Deep squat
- Hurdle step
- In-line lunge
- Shoulder mobility
- Active straight-leg raise
- Trunk stability push-up
- Rotary stability

The FMS screens mobility and stability patterns of fundamental human movement. It's simple and reliable.

The FMS is beyond the scope of this book, but it's a tool I use that has great value in screening movement and identifying potential gaps.

Remember, it's a screen for potential issues, not a test or assessment.

To learn more about it, go to **FunctionalMovement.com** – and if you really want to understand movement on a deep level, you must check out Gray Cook's great book *Movement.*

THE SITTING-RISING TEST

The Sitting-Rising Test (SRT) is an amazing movement test designed by a Brazilian doctor.

It's simple, reliable, and has significant prognostic value.

Here's how the test works.

Without worrying about speed of movement, try to sit down on the floor and then rise back up, using the minimum amount of support you need to sit to rise.

A picture is worth a thousand words, so when you have a chance, google "sitting rising test" to see how simple but challenging this is.

You'll be able to see how the test measures strength/power, coordination, flexibility, balance, and other physical qualities.

While this test has been studied in older individuals (ages 51-80), I'm sure you can see how something like this can be a valuable assessment tool for anyone, regardless of age.

As with previous studies covered earlier, the poorer the performance, the less favorable outcomes patients had. Specifically, low scores on the SRT were associated with a greater than six-fold higher incidence of mortality in men and women.

GAIT

Observing how we walk is another valuable observational tool.

Gait analysis is one of those detailed assessments that go beyond the scope of this book, but it's something I frequently use as an indicator of quality movement.

For example, I just happen to recently observe someone demonstrating excessive side bending (or lateral trunk flexion) as they walked.

Why?

Weak hip abductors.

Once again, you may not be trained to look for dysfunctions in gait mechanics, but anyone can look at gait and see if any gross motor deficits or observational dysfunctions are present.

Look at the big picture.

You can even video yourself. Check out what you notice about your gait, and you might be surprised.

Here are some examples of what to look for:
- Spine posture, position, and displacement of the upper body
- Arm movement (or lack of)
- Hip range of motion or muscle weakness
- Knee range of motion
- Ankle range of motion
- Foot position (toe out, toe in, supination, excessive pronation)
- Cadence or speed of walking
- Unusual movements, patterns, or compensations

The simple observation of how you walk can be extremely revealing.

If you really want to better understand gait analysis, 2 great books are *Born to Walk* by James Earls and *What the Foot* by my friend Gary Ward

(who I have interviewed on episodes #97 and #98 of **The Rdella Training®
Podcast**).

CATEGORIES OF MOVEMENT

This is something Dan John has been talking about for a while now, and it's important.

Basically, these are "categories" of fundamental movement that can be assessed, as well as trained.

What I mean is that each category can be used to assess movement.

And, each category is also a way to train.

The movements listed below can also consist of different variations as you'll see.

The great thing about these categories is that they are all valuable movements, which is why they are so essential for strength and performance.

Let's review the essential movement categories.

PUSH

A push movement is what is sounds like – a push or a press of some kind.

It can include a push-up, an overhead press, a bench press, a jerk, or any number of pushing movements.

PULL

A pull is also what it sounds like – a pulling motion.

The classic example is a pull-up, although there are other variations of pulls such as rows or even deadlifts, where you are pulling the weight up from the floor.

Not to confuse the matter, but the deadlift is also a hinge and you could argue it's a push movement.

We can debate why it could be categorized as each, but just realize that complex movements like deadlifts have elements of each.

HINGE

Whereas the first two were easy to guess, most people are unaware of this one.

A hinge is a movement that occurs at the hips.

The hips fold, and the spine is kept straight or in neutral.

You are hinging at the hips to gain the movement.

A hinge is athletic and functional.

It's different from a squat because the hip motion (or hinging) is the dominant movement.

Hinge = movement at the hips

Squat = movement at the hips and knees

The best example of the hinge is the kettlebell swing, where the kettlebell is projected horizontally through an efficient hinge pattern.

As mentioned, the deadlift is also considered a hinge movement because of the folding at the hips.

SQUAT

We all know what a squat is, yet many people struggle with it.

There are many variations of the squat, including:

- Barbell back squat
- Front squat
- Zercher squat
- Bodyweight squat
- Pistol squat
- Overhead squat
- Goblet squat
- Double kettlebell front squat

Many of the squat variations are effective and useful depending on the goal and the individual.

A good squat always begins with the demonstration of a high-quality bodyweight squat, then progresses from there.

If you can't "air squat" or bodyweight squat properly, you probably shouldn't load the movement with weight.

The squat is critically important for optimal function and athleticism, as you and I know.

CARRY

Thanks to Dan John and Dr. Stuart McGill for enlightening us on the value of the **loaded carry.**

There's no magic to performing this exercise.

The magic seems to be in what it does for us.

Most people don't do carries, although they are becoming more recognized in strength and conditioning communities these days.

A carry is simply picking up a heavy object (a kettlebell is a great example) and going for a walk with it.

Farmer's walks, suitcase carries, and waiter's walks are examples of loaded carries.

The stability, postural demand, strength, and conditioning is exceptional as you walk for a distance with the weight.

Carries usually start out easy, but no one would ever describe carries as being easy after a long walk.

If they are not challenging, your weight is too light.

Loaded carries are a simple, extremely high-value exercise. For more on carries, read any of the great work by Dan John.

GROUND WORK

The perfect example of ground work is the Turkish Get-Up (TGU).

The TGU is a magnificent movement for health and performance.

We'll cover the TGU in detail later as it's a key kettlebell exercise, but for now just know that the TGU is one of the most valuable human movements we have.

Why?

Because it requires movement from the floor to a tall standing position and then back down again.

The day we lose the ability to get up and down from the floor is a very bad day.

Additional movements include crawling and rolling, which I'll cover later, as well.

All the specifics of using these movements for strength training exercises will be covered in Section IV.

The most important thing is to understand your baseline of movement and make sure to establish good movement patterns before adding loads.

Now you know there are many ways to assess and improve movement.

What if you don't have good movement?

We'll get to that in Chapter 11.

Many things taught in this book will help to improve it, as you'll see.

Next, we move to another important topic to understand before developing (or redeveloping) your training program.

CHAPTER 8: THE 7 LAWS

"Fitness is not about being better than someone else.
It's about being better than you used to be."
–Unknown

The secret to a great training approach has more to do with the laws it follows as opposed to the training program itself.

Well, laws and principles.

All training programs work.

Ok, maybe not all, but most.

That is, they will work to develop strength as long as they are built on these laws and fundamental principles.

That said, all programs don't work forever, and some programs are much more effective than others.

And you need to understand how to build strength to recognize how and why strength plateaus.

The iconic Dr. Fred Hatfield has discussed the vital importance of the 7 laws of training in his outstanding work.

These are so important that we'll review each one, then discuss how we can successfully apply these to training.

LAW #1: THE LAW OF INDIVIDUAL DIFFERENCES

We are all different, and everyone has different strengths and weakness. Because of this, no program fits all individuals.

There is no single "best" program for all of us.

We are all built differently, from structure to function.

This means that our techniques could vary, our movement patterns could be slightly different, and our endurance capacities could differ greatly among individuals.

We are all built differently, and each of us is a physiologically unique individual.

The law of individual differences is a major consideration in all training programs, which is why we must approach them from an individualistic standpoint.

LAW #2: THE OVERCOMPENSATION PRINCIPLE

The human body reacts to stress and overcompensates to handle that stress.

In other words, we adapt to our training over time.

Beginners will see the greatest advancement in training benefits as these adaptations occur to a much greater extent. There are simply more challenges to adapt to in a shorter period of time.

Good news to those of you reading this who are new to the iron game.

On the other hand, the advanced or experienced lifter will see only incremental progress in their training methods as they are much more "adapted" to training.

LAW #3: THE OVERLOAD PRINCIPLE

This is progressive overload as we've touched on previously in Chapter 3: Important Terms and Concepts.

This principle states that we must progressively load the body with greater weight or place greater demands to our training to achieve benefit.

This is how we make progress: with increases in training variables.

Training variables such as:

- volume
- intensity
- duration
- frequency
- skills

However, we cannot train like this indefinitely.

Consequences will be burnout, plateau, regression, or injury.

This is where a periodized approach comes into play and specific periods of de-loading are necessary.

LAW #4: THE SPECIFIC ADAPTATION TO IMPOSED DEMAND (S.A.I.D.) PRINCIPLE

The principle states that you must impose demands specific to the desired goals.

If the goal is to increase speed, then you focus your efforts on speed training and related progressions.

If the goal is to increase hypertrophy, then you progressively increase volume or other variables specific to hypertrophy training.

And, if the goal is to increase maximum strength with powerlifting, then you progressively increase the demands of intensity and specificity for powerlifting.

To meet the training goal, you apply more demands specific to the goal.

The SAID principle is critical to understand and apply in an effective programming approach.

LAW #5: THE USE/DISUSE PRINCIPLE AND LAW OF REVERSIBILITY

This is an interesting law because it is essentially stating that we use it or lose it.

This means that if we fail to train a specific skill or series of skills, we will lose the efficiency of those skills over time.

Again, use it or lose it. But, here's what's also interesting about this law.

If we have obtained a skill or skills and they have been lost due to disuse, it's much easier to regain those skills if we begin to re-train them.

Think of learning to ride a bike. Once we learn, our nervous system always remembers that skill or motor program. This is the **muscle memory** phenomenon. When we have previously learned a skill, the relearning process happens more rapidly than it took to initially gain that skill.

If we have learned something from a neurological level, it's much easier to regain that skill, even if we have not engaged in it for an extended period of time.

LAW #6: THE SPECIFICITY PRINCIPLE

"Do the thing, and you will have the power."
–Ralph Waldo Emerson

To get better at a task, we must do that thing, not do a hundred other things.

This is similar to the SAID principle. However, while the SAID principle is about imposing the demand, this law is about specificity of the skill.

To get better at kettlebell swings, you do kettlebell swings.

To get better and stronger with deadlifts, you deadlift.

As you prepare for a powerlifting meet, your training would become more specialized or specific to the powerlifts with accessory work diminishing.

The law simply states that if you want to get better at something, you focus on that thing.

As we saw with the 5 levels of strength, specificity is extremely important for skill development.

LAW #7: THE GENERAL ADAPTATION SYNDROME

This principle contains 3 important stages or phases that encompass training. These occur when you begin a new training program.

1. ALARM.

The alarm stage is the **initial stage** when the body reacts to training stress. Let's say when you begin a new training program, for example. Remember the overload principle.

2. RESISTANCE.

This is the stage when the body begins to **adapt** to increased demands of stress. Remember the overcompensation principle.

3. EXHAUSTION.

This is a fine line that states if we continue to train at a high level, eventually we'll be forced to stop as negative outcomes (e.g., injury, overreaching, overtraining) may result.

This syndrome has been revised and renamed the **fitness-fatigue model.**

Differences will be notable between novice and advanced athletes.

More **advanced athletes** or lifters will be able to endure more because of the laws of overload and overcompensation.

Novice athletes – although they will be able to elicit far greater training benefits – will exhaust must faster and will need more recovery due to the alarm stage.

All of this will depend on the first law, the law of individual differences.

HOW TO USE THESE LAWS

What should we do with this information? If you do nothing with the information you just learned, it's meaningless.

We should use these principles holistically and apply them to our programming and training.

Let me explain.

We may have different goals, backgrounds, and abilities, and this is why **there is no "best" program** for everyone – just like there is no "best diet."

There are general principles for optimal nutrition, but to say there is a "best" way to eat would be inaccurate.

There are many great programs, and there are certainly crappy ones.

But it's important to realize that we are all different, and we may have to scale programs to meet our goals and individual backgrounds.

Scale: To adjust or modify a program according to our "uniqueness," individuality, training background, and skills.

By fully understanding and applying these laws, we'll have far better short – and long-term training success.

- Understand and apply these laws
- Commit them to memory
- Post them on a wall
- Store them in your phone

Do whatever you need to do to remember them so you can build your training with these laws in mind.

The next chapter will be different than anything you've ever read before, taking the concept of physical strength beyond muscles.

How does strength improve overall health?

CHAPTER 9: A SYSTEMS APPROACH TO STRENGTH

"Much of what we call aging is nothing more than
the accumulation of a lifetime of inactivity.
Muscles shrink. Body fat increases.
The results are an increased risk of
diabetes, hypertension, and osteoporosis"
–Dr. William Evans

In terms of optimizing your health – this information is critical. It's a way of approaching strength that you've likely never heard before.

In this chapter, I'll show you how **strength equals wellness.**

You and I are going to look at the relationship of strength on each of the systems in the human body.

In some sense, I hope this information motivates you even more to use strength training at a higher level.

It's important for each of us to really understand the impact of strength training, specifically how strength improves our health.

And, what are the devastating consequences of lacking strength or failing to train as we age?

This information was born out of many conversations I've had with top fitness experts and also noticing the gaps in the literature addressing the topic of strength and health.

I've already said **strength training is our fountain of youth.** Now I'll explain why in this chapter.

If there is such a thing as a magic bullet to optimize human health, strength training would be it.

A systems approach to the human body exposes countless new ways to envision how strength improves physical potential.

This is an area that's almost never discussed but long-term health may be the most important benefit of getting stronger.

Recently, I heard something that was really interesting.

In a podcast interview I was listening to, I heard an extremely smart physician discussing the benefits of exercise (by the way, this doc is also an athlete, so I know he gets it).

He was being asked about exercise and what he thought was the most important form of exercise.

Care to guess what his response was?

Heavy strength training.

The brilliant doctor stated that **many of our problems are a result of our inability to be strong.**

We are de-conditioned at the muscular level.

The theme of this entire book is that we need to continually build strength because we lose it as we age. That is, we'll lose muscle unless we do everything we can to slow the decline.

As we age, we will invariably lose strength at a certain point in our lives no matter what we do. However, we can prevent the decline as much as possible to extend our strength and be the best we can be today and into the future.

Even if we were "stronger" when we were younger, we are still preventing the decline and being our best version of ourselves by training with the goal of becoming strong.

Strength training contributes to health and longevity, as well as function and performance.

Some of the health benefits of resistance exercise include:

- Increased resting metabolic rate
- Improved glucose metabolism
- Improved blood lipid profiles
- Decreased gastrointestinal transit time (reduces the risk of colon cancer)
- Reduces resting blood pressure
- Improved bone mineral density
- Reduced pain and discomfort from arthritic conditions
- Reduction in low back pain
- Enhanced mobility and flexibility
- Improved maximal aerobic capacity

To better understand how we gain these benefits, let's take a look at the systems of the body. And, in all fairness, I am going look at each and every one.

THE 12 SYSTEMS OF THE HUMAN BODY

1. THE INTEGUMENTARY SYSTEM
2. THE SKELETAL SYSTEM
3. THE MUSCULAR SYSTEM
4. THE LYMPHATIC SYSTEM
5. THE IMMUNE SYSTEM
6. THE RESPIRATORY SYSTEM
7. THE NERVOUS SYSTEM
8. THE ENDOCRINE SYSTEM
9. THE CARDIOVASCULAR SYSTEM
10. THE DIGESTIVE SYSTEM
11. THE URINARY SYSTEM
12. THE REPRODUCTIVE SYSTEM

And, we can debate one other system although it's not recognized as a true system of the human body.

That system is...

THE FASCIAL SYSTEM

We'll discuss the fascial system last.

This chapter has become my personal quest to better understand how strength training impacts our entire body beyond our muscular and nervous systems.

The genesis of this topic came from a podcast interview I had with Dr. Fred Hatfield. "Dr. Squat," as he is often called, is legendary for his contributions not only as a strength athlete, but world-renowned expert in strength training, bodybuilding, and performance enhancement.

If you'd like to check out the interviews I had with Dr. Hatfield, be sure to listen to **The Rdella Training® Podcast** in iTunes.

Dr. Hatfield made a statement during one of our conversations and said something along the lines of "how does strength affect health?"

I thought a lot about that question ever since, and what you'll see here is my answer.

We're going to look at each of the body's 12 systems.

After briefly covering each system, I'll provide the verdict as to whether strength training would have any impact on that system in the human body.

Let's take a quick look.

INTEGUMENTARY SYSTEM

The integumentary system consists of our skin, nails, and hair.

It would be a stretch to say that strength contributes to this system in any meaningful way.

Although I do see how movement stimulates other systems (such as endocrine) that may indirectly contribute to skin health, we can't say there's a direct link between the integumentary system and strength training.

Verdict: NO

SKELETAL SYSTEM

The skeletal system is composed of 206 bones in the adult human body.

There is no question that resistance exercise builds stronger bones and contributes to increased bone mineral density (BMD).

Increased BMD helps prevent fractures, especially those that become prevalent in women (or men) who develop osteoporosis or osteopenia.

The improvement of bone health is a major and undisputed benefit of resistance exercise.

Verdict: YES

MUSCULAR SYSTEM

There are hundreds of skeletal muscles in the human body, not to mention cardiac muscle and smooth muscle.

The impact of strength training is most obvious to the muscular system in the following ways:

- develops strength
- builds muscular hypertrophy
- improves muscle tissue quality
- stimulates muscle physiology
- improves rates of muscle firing and activity
- enhances mitochondrial function

The reason most of us train is to get stronger and develop the muscular system to its fullest.

And, as you know by now, sarcopenia is the progressive loss of muscle tissue as we age.

We have to do everything we can to slow down this age-related muscle loss.

Verdict: YES

LYMPHATIC SYSTEM

The lymphatic system is basically a filtration system that filters debris and toxins from our blood vessels.

It's also the housing station for our white blood cells, which are extremely important to fight disease and illness.

Exercise and movement help to stimulate the fluid and drainage of the lymphatic system.

In other words, when we move more, the lymphatic system works better.

When we are more sedentary, the lymphatic system needs to work harder.

More movement means improved efficiency of the lymphatic system because it helps the filtration process.

Verdict: YES

IMMUNE SYSTEM

The immune system is a functional system that protects the body via immune responses.

It is compromised of the spleen, thymus, lymph nodes, and bone marrow.

This amazing and important system is strengthened by being active and exercising.

Too much exercise, however, can be detrimental and overly stress the immune system.

This can occur in states of overreaching or overtraining.

Verdict: YES

RESPIRATORY SYSTEM

The respiratory system (our lungs) is the center for our ability to breathe properly and efficiently.

This system keeps blood supplied with oxygen and thereby removes carbon dioxide from our system.

The respiratory system is our ability to have efficient gas exchange for high performance and for daily living.

Depending on the type of resistance exercise you do and providing you have learned to breathe or ventilate properly, strength training will certainly improve the function and performance of the respiratory system.

Metabolic conditioning (MetCon) exercise and protocols –for example, high-intensity interval training (HIIT) – has been shown to improve aerobic capacity.

Verdict: YES

NERVOUS SYSTEM

The nervous system consists of the brain, spinal cord, and peripheral nerves. These are 2 distinct systems known as the central nervous system (CNS) and peripheral nervous system (PNS).

The brain and spinal cord are the CNS, and everything else in the nervous system belongs to the PNS.

Strength training is truly a neurological process in which the nervous system is stimulated to a high degree to recruit motor units, which we've covered previously.

Strength, movement, motor control, myelination, and technical proficiency are developed through processes in the nervous system.

Verdict: YES

ENDOCRINE SYSTEM

The endocrine system is composed of many glands that secrete hormones, such as:

- growth hormone (GH)
- testosterone (T)
- insulin (I)
- insulin-like growth factor (IGF)
- cortisol (C)
- brain-derived neurotropic factor (BDNF)

The hormonal response to exercise is quite overwhelming as many favorable hormonal changes occur during, after, and as a result of resistance exercise training.

These hormonal responses significantly contribute to:

- improved body composition changes
- improved strength
- anti-aging benefits
- improved energy and well-being
- prevention of many major life-threatening diseases (cardiovascular disease, diabetes, and certain types of cancer)

Verdict: YES

CARDIOVASCULAR SYSTEM

The cardiovascular system is composed of the heart and all circulatory tissues (arteries and veins).

Depending on the training variables implemented in a training program, the cardiovascular system can be positively influenced.

For example, when MetCon or HIIT are incorporated, the cardiovascular benefits are outstanding.

On the other hand, if you're doing maximal strength programming (i.e., a powerlifting program) there will be less of an effect on the cardiovascular system.

Strength training can improve the function of the cardiovascular system, depending on the training variables that are used in the program.

Verdict: YES

DIGESTIVE SYSTEM

The digestive system breaks down the food we eat to enter into the bloodstream to distribute to the cells for energy and nutrients. Waste by-products are eliminated.

The practice of regular exercise has been found to improve the digestion and elimination process. In a small research study, it was reported that GI (gastrointestinal) transit time was accelerated in middle-aged and older men who performed strength training.

The significance of this is a reduction in colon cancer.

Granted the study was small, but it was meaningful data on the influence of strength training on the digestive system.

And, certainly the combination of exercise training and optimal nutrition will enhance the performance of the digestive system.

We don't train to improve our digestive system function, but there certainly seems to be benefits to this system as a result.

Interesting stuff, huh?

Verdict: YES

URINARY SYSTEM

The urinary system eliminates excess nitrogen from the body. It also regulates water, electrolyte, and acid-base balance in the body.

Does strength training impact the urinary system in any way?

Honestly, I don't think it matters. At least I have not found any evidence to support such a claim.

What could impact this system would be the hydration and electrolyte replenishment that's involved in hard strength training, but not so much the training itself.

Verdict: NO

REPRODUCTIVE

Obviously, the reproductive system is different for males and females. Regardless, this is an interesting system as it relates to strength and exercise.

Indirectly, you could argue that there is an impact on sex-related hormones (testosterone for males, estrogen for females) as a result of strength training, which then does have an impact on the reproductive system and sex drive.

Verdict: YES

THE FASCIAL SYSTEM

Now, let's discuss that "other" system.

The fascial system is a body-wide tensional network of connective tissue. This connective tissue, called fascia, is fibrous in nature and is shaped by tensile strain as opposed to compression.

There is emerging science in the area of training the fascial system and understanding the role it has on the human body and performance.

Human movement and many forms of physical training have a major impact on the fascial system, which helps to organize the fascia for optimal movement, function, and the prevention of injuries.

The fascial system is an amazing topic and goes beyond the scope of this book, but it's worth mentioning here as we examine systems of the human body.

Sports science is embracing the study of fascia. And, strength training definitely impacts the fascial system.

There are many fascinating books, articles, and scientific publications on the influence of physical training and fascia. *Fascia in Sport and Movement* by Robert Schleip specifically looks at the effects of kettlebell training and other training methods on the fascial system.

SUMMARY OF THE SYSTEMS APPROACH

Out of the systems in the human body we've reviewed (including the fascia system), potentially 11 out of 13 systems are directly influenced by strength training.

11 OUT OF 13 SYSTEMS IN THE HUMAN BODY ARE POSITIVELY IMPACTED BY STRENGTH TRAINING.

That is significant!

This is overwhelming evidence when you consider the impact of strength training on total-body health.

Now, we must understand there are many variables to consider with this statement such as type of strength, type of programming, and training variables used.

In general, strength has a major effect on our body that greatly contributes to our overall level of health.

And, the information is this **systems approach** doesn't include how strength improves our daily functional capacity – our ability to perform better each day just by increasing levels of strength.

The fact is that we need to be strength training for the rest of our lives (as long as we are physically able).

Without strength, we're simply not operating at our full potential.

CHAPTER 10: MORE THAN STRONG

"I am the master of my fate: I am the captain of my soul"
–Invictus by William Ernest Henley

I'd never claim that strength is the only thing we need, but strength is our foundation.

What are you trying to achieve?

Almost no matter what that is, strength will help.

What specific goals are you looking to achieve with your training?

Once you know the goal, the goal dictates the programming approach.

Focus on the **one big thing** at a time. This is what gets me results. It keeps me focused, keeps me moving forward, and I have fun.

When I chase too many things, it usually doesn't get me anywhere.

ONE BIG THING	Programming Examples
FAT LOSS	Metabolic Conditioning
MAXIMUM STRENGTH	Powerlifting
MUSCLE BUILDING	Volume Training, Targeted Training Approach
PERFORMANCE GOAL	Olympic weightlifting
OPTIMAL HEALTH	GPP approach, focus on fundamentals

These are just examples, and we'll cover how to clarify exactly what you want very soon.

As we're talking about goals and getting clear on things, I want to talk about other physical qualities beyond just strength.

One of my major influences is the legendary Dr. Fred Hatfield, who stated:

"There is no such thing as a fit individual."

Let's clarify what this means because I don't want it to be misunderstood.

We cannot achieve maximum proficiency with multiple physical qualities – ALL at once.

When one quality goes up, another quality goes down.

We cannot simultaneously have the highest levels of strength, endurance, power, agility, speed, and conditioning. Something has to give.

What makes an elite powerlifter does not make an elite sprinter. We cannot run in a marathon and at the same time compete in Olympic weightlifting.

This is critical to understand, especially in today's extreme fitness climate.

Yes, **we can have general levels of many different qualities at once,** but the reality is that they will be relatively low levels. We can do a lot of things at a low level.

According to Dan John, this is Quadrant 3 in his 4 Quadrants approach.

Here's an overview of his model:

QUADRANT 1 = Lots of qualities at a very LOW level

Physical education class and broadly organized activities. The truest GPP approach we have.

QUADRANT 2 = Lots of qualities at a HIGH level

Collision sports and occupations. This is professional athletes and tactical personnel.

QUADRANT 3 = Few qualities at a LOW or MODERATE level

According to Dan, this is where most people are, in Quadrant 3.

QUADRANT 4 = Few (or one) qualities at the highest level

This is the International Olympic weightlifter or elite powerlifter, for example.

We all fall into 1 of these 4 quadrants, most of us being in Quadrant 3.

This method can help you decide what you want most: to be a generalist or a specialist. This is not to say we can't retain other qualities aside from our current goal, just that we can't excel in everything at once.

IMPORTANT QUALITIES BESIDES STRENGTH

With that in mind, let's take a look at important qualities outside of strength. The qualities we need or want will depend on our goals and functional objectives.

Besides strength, other important qualities I'll discuss are:

- Movement and Motor Control
- Power
- Endurance
- Speed
- Agility
- Flexibility
- Mobility
- Balance
- Aesthetics
- Health

MOVEMENT AND MOTOR CONTROL

Again, we have to start with good movement and having a baseline of quality movement, but what is that exactly?

By definition, it's the act, process, or result of moving. Yet, it goes beyond that.

Good movement is the ability to demonstrate full mobility, stability, and motor control through full range of motion with safe and proper biomechanics of the specific demand.

Movement should be dynamic, free-form, fluid, and graceful. It's a combination of motor control, mobility, and stability.

Does strength help movement?

Absolutely.

Motor control (neuromuscular coordination) is the process by which humans and animals use their neuromuscular system to activate and coordinate the muscles and limbs in the performance of a motor skill.

A motor skill is movement.

We already discussed the importance of quality human movement, and depending on the type of training method, strength training will improve neuromuscular coordination.

For athletes and recreational exercisers, motor control is extremely important. I would argue that we all need to be "better movers" and improve our motor control skills so that we function at the highest level.

This book is about being the best version of ourselves. The training methods discussed will help us to move better, move with precision and grace, and optimize our bodies for peak performance.

This applies whether for sport or simply the challenges of daily living. Strength training significantly impacts our nervous system and our motor control.

The Edge of Strength is a movement-based approach that improves motor control so that we become better movers and better performers.

POWER

As we've covered, **power is the ability to produce force rapidly.**

We covered why it's important to develop the quality of power for athletic performance, as well as function.

The longer we can maintain this quality, the more functional and high performing we will be in our lives.

Please refer back to Chapter 6 (Strength Science) if you need to refresh this important concept.

ENDURANCE

When you think of endurance athlete, what comes to mind?

For most, it's the image of a marathon runner.

The truth is that endurance is a physical quality that goes beyond just aerobic capacity. There is aerobic endurance, muscular endurance, and even mental endurance (or mental toughness).

We can define **endurance as the ability to perform a task over time.** Endurance is multi-faceted, and training for it as a primary goal can be comprehensive.

That said, strength can greatly impact endurance.

For example, there is evidence that heavy resistance exercise improves the running economy in distance runners..

SPEED

For sports, speed is highly regarded. Many would even say "speed is king," not strength.

This may be true, depending on the sport.

But, even those coaches who champion speed would agree that strength is still foundational for any high-performing athlete.

Speed – a function of **fast-twitch muscle fibers** and biomechanical factors – is a highly valued quality for physical excellence, but it's totally dependent on the sport.

While the potential for speed has been considered primarily genetic or inherited, recent evidence has proven that speed can be enhanced or trained with specific and proper training.

In other words, we can learn to run faster (improve our motor control), and we can develop **strength speed** by training for strength.

AGILITY

Agility is the ability to change direction rapidly. This is dependent on speed, strength, and balance.

Agility is task-specific and can be improved with practice, proper training, and experience.

It's most important for athleticism. Both aerobic fitness and muscular endurance are important to maintain agility.

Strength training, or course, will be a contributing factor to the development of agility.

FLEXIBILITY AND MOBILITY

Flexibility and mobility are different things, although they are often used synonymously.

Flexibility refers to the length of muscle tissues, whereas mobility refers to how well joints move.

Flexibility = movement as related to muscle tissue

Mobility = movement as related to the joints

If we have limited movement, for example, we may find that our muscles are tight or inflexible or that our joints are immobile and restricted.

Not to confuse the matter, but limited movement could also be a motor control or stability issue.

Strength training, certainly the methods in this book, helps to improve, restore, or maintain flexibility and mobility.

Mobility has rightfully received much more attention lately and has become an entire entity in fitness and performance today.

What I've found is that the strength training methods I advocate in this book have greatly contributed to my mobility – far greater than I would have ever imagined.

AESTHETICS

I'm mentioning aesthetics because we all want to look good. No matter what the fitness goal, we all want to look more athletic.

Everybody wants to lose fat and build muscle.

Whether you're training for the primary, secondary, or tertiary goals of aesthetics – appearance is usually part of the equation in most people's training objectives.

In the introduction of this book, I mentioned that this was this my primary training goal for many years when I was a competitive bodybuilder. While my goals have significantly changed, aesthetics are still in the mix.

Is there any better method to change our physique than with strength training?

Focusing on "cardio" isn't doing anything to build muscle.

And, we've covered why we all need muscle.

HEALTH

We covered this is in great detail in the last chapter.

We covered how strength training impacts the different systems of the human body.

Now, keep in mind, health and fitness are two distinct things, although they're often used interchangeably.

Health is maintaining a disease-free state; fitness is the ability to perform a task.

You can be very fit but not healthy and vice versa.

For example, you can be a high-level weightlifter but be affected by a chronic illness or be generally "unhealthy." And, you can have a level of peak health, but not be very strong for powerlifting or weightlifting.

Health and fitness are not always mutually exclusive.

Ideally, if you perform strength training appropriately and strategically, you'll reap the benefits of both.

CHAPTER 11: BECOMING BULLETPROOF

"Strength fixes almost everything."
–Mark Reifkind

Becoming bulletproof is about avoiding injury and performing at a high level over a long period of time.

Who wouldn't want to do that?

I've had this concept in mind – to become bulletproof – long before reading the great work of Tim Anderson, who also discussed this concept in a similar way.

He defines being bulletproof as having a healthy body that allows us to enjoy life well into the golden years.

Who says at 70 or 80 years old we should be broke and limited in our functional capacity?

Becoming bulletproof is about being resilient and training smarter to prevent injuries from occurring in the first place.

I take injury prevention very seriously for a few reasons.

- **My own experience sustaining an injury**
- **My background as a physical therapist**
- **For the long-term training approach to optimize health and performance**

Now, I want to share my personal story about the importance of injury prevention with you.

I learned many valuable lessons that changed my life, but I did it the hard way.

MY INJURED BACK

I was 19 years old when it happened, soon after my first bodybuilding competition.

I placed 3rd that year, which was a great debut for me considering the guys who placed ahead of me were pretty swole, as I recall.

I was training very intensely at the time with **no concept of injury prevention,** I was on a mission in the gym. I was a hardcore bodybuilder, putting all my energy and focus into bodybuilding.

I literally lived and breathed bodybuilding, and I had lofty aspirations about my future after that show.

One day, lifting a heavy barbell up from the floor, I was doing heavy barbell shrugs.

I should have been in a squat rack doing this, but I was lifting the loaded, heavy bar up from the floor to do shrugs (*mistake #1*).

While it's hard to specifically remember, I'm sure I had crappy technique deadlifting the bar up from the floor (*mistake #2*).

I felt a "pop" in my back.

Although I didn't think much of it at the time, I knew something was wrong.

Later that night, my back was hurting badly.

Never having experienced a major injury before, I figured it was just a muscle strain and that I'd be fine in a couple of days (*mistake #3*).

The next day or so later, I went to the gym for leg day, ignoring the pain in my low back.

Guess what I did?

Back squats (*mistake #4*).

Needless to say, that was a stupid thing to do. The pain progressively increased and was radiating in my left leg. It wasn't long after that I was immobile and in constant pain. It went downhill fast from there.

The truth is I was young and dumb.

I ignored the signals my body was telling me because, no matter what, *I had to lift.*

Let me recap the mistakes so you can learn from them:

1. Did something I shouldn't have done (*shrugs off the floor*)
2. Used poor technique
3. Ignored the pain
4. Did not modify or adjust training

I ended up having a severely **herniated L4-5 disc with radiculopathy** (radiating pain into the left leg).

The injury occurred in May.

I had the surgery in July.

It all happened so fast, but I'll never forget that experience.

This injury seemed like the worst thing imaginable, but over time, it came to be the best thing that ever happened to me.

I learned a very valuable lesson that I've implemented for decades now.

The lesson is **LISTEN TO YOUR BODY** and never ignore pain. I'll talk more about pain as an indicator in a minute.

After the surgery, the rehab and physical therapy were a very long process. My goal was to come back and compete in bodybuilding.

I competed again approximately 2 years after I sustained the injury.

How's my back today?

Strong, powerful, and healthy.

I attribute my back health today to the kettlebell and barbell training I do, which I'll discuss in detail in Section IV.

As a matter of fact, the only time my back does bother me at all is when I take off training for an extended period of time.

That leads me to this concept of *"becoming bulletproof."*

How I was training at 19 was not going to help me gain *The Edge of Strength*.

While there are some dramatic and exciting things happening in the fitness industry today, there are also some very disheartening and foolish things going as well.

Extreme workouts where you push past your physical limitations – in regards to safety – will not help you become bulletproof.

There's no more accurate term to prevent or minimize the risk for injury than becoming bulletproof and that's why I love and respect this concept.

There is absolutely no guarantee that you will be 100% free from injury as you engage in physical training.

But, you can greatly reduce the incidence of injuries by implementing the following strategies and by using an intelligent approach to short-term and long-term training.

We all need to train safe, period.

KEY COMPONENTS OF SAFE TRAINING

We've already discussed the importance of establishing quality movement. Even if we have quality movement, we need to always work to improve it.

If we don't have it, then we need to work on fixing our "weak links" as best we can through corrective exercises or uncomplicated programming approaches.

Here's a little tough love, though.

Not all things are fixable or correctable.

What I mean is that if you have an old injury that limits your movement and mobility, you may not be able to fix it due to chronic tissue or joint changes.

If you have a structural problem, such as scoliosis, you're not likely to fix it with a corrective exercise.

This is something to keep in mind and not lead your training in the direction of false expectations.

With that said, **we must focus on quality of movement** as best we can in all that we do.

We must do the best we can with what we've got.

PAIN IS AN INDICATOR

If you have pain and think you can work through it, you're making a mistake.

Pain is a signal, an indicator that something is wrong.

There are different kinds of pain, but I'm generally referring to trying to train and work through an existing injury because you don't want to stop training.

If you have pain and are trying to work through it, you really have 2 training choices:

1 – Stop Training (*If pain is exacerbated as a result of training)

This is the hardest thing for most of us – to stop training.

Anyone that is into their training doesn't want to be told to stop going and lose momentum.

If everything hurts and makes things worse, there is no option other than to stop, although some exercises could actually be therapeutic. If that's the case...

2 – Do Only What Does Not Induce Symptoms (Pain-free training)

It should go without saying, but if you have pain, you need to seek out a qualified health care provider.

Please get medical help if you have an injury, and don't mess around at the gym if something is going on.

Pain changes everything. If you can find what you can do without provoking pain, this would be a reasonable approach. If you do something, and it hurts – don't continue to do it!

It's pretty simple, yet it's also surprising how many people try to work through their injuries only to make them worse.

I'd include myself in that group in the past, but it's a valuable **lesson learned.** Now I'll never make that mistake again.

So, how do you become bulletproof to reduce the risk of injuries you'll have to work around?

CHECK YOUR EGO

It's important to not let your ego get the best of you by motivating you to try to push through injuries.

Have the courage to get medical help, take time off, or re-adjust your training altogether. Do what you need to do to get through a bad situation without making things worse.

Let's say you're in a workshop or similar group training experience, and you get sucked into going for a PR with something maybe you're not quite ready for yet.

But, you go for it anyway because of the peer pressure and the situation you're in. We've all been there and been in situations like this.

Sometimes there are parts of workshops, seminars, training events, or workout sessions that are planned to push people to go for new PRs.

I've experienced it myself, and it's fine if you're ready for it.

If you aren't ready, check your ego.

Don't let the spirit of the situation coax your ego to take over and get you into trouble. It's not worth it.

Know what you can do and cannot do, and don't get caught up in the moment. Peer pressure is not a good reason to go for a new PR.

If you go for new PRs, you better damn well make sure you're ready to test a new PR.

GET COACHING

Even coaches need coaches.

Dan John told me something along those lines during an interview in a podcast session. Dan is a "coach's coach." So if he has a coach, you and I need one too.

Don't kid yourself. We all need coaches because a great coach makes you better. A great coach will improve your technical proficiency in the skills I outline in this book. A great coach will keep us moving forward and keep our focus on training safe.

Whether you work with a coach once a year, once a month, or once a week, find a great coach.

It may be the most important investment you make in yourself.

DON'T BE OVERCOME BY FEAR

While we need to train smart and be sensible, **we don't want to be so risk averse that we're afraid to lift heavy weights.**

Heavy weight is instructive – to a point.

We don't want to be fearful of heavy lifting. We want to be smart about heavy lifting. There is a difference. This means putting the weight down when technique starts to deteriorate.

Is it one more rep even worth it if your technique sucks?

I don't think so.

There's a fine line here, but you have to learn when enough is enough.

Heavy weight teaches us much more about movement and optimal biomechanics than light weight does.

To become bulletproof and be the best versions of ourselves, we do need to train heavy. But heavy strength training requires proper progression, coaching, and technique.

You just need to be smart about it.

TECHNIQUE AND SKILL DEVELOPMENT

Let's revisit the 1% rule.

It should be painfully obvious – the better our skills and techniques, the safer our training will be.

Yet, how many people approach their training session with the idea to make progress, to become better today than they were yesterday?

I'm not sure, but I know it's the minority. That's because it requires focusing on long-term progress and not just short-term gratification.

The 1% RULE is a simple but brilliant strategy for long-term results. It is about focusing on getting just a little bit better each and every training session.

Improve every day by 1%, and be a little better today than you were yesterday.

This is a little **mindset hack** to keep us moving forward.

Always work on skill development and technique to become bullet-proof. It's a simple approach that goes a long way.

EMBRACE RATIONALISM

This is one of my favorite concepts to practice in the long-term fitness approach and culminates from concepts we've already covered.

Be rational in everything you do.

Don't rush into decisions when it comes to strength training and going for the next level.

When you train, ask yourself the following questions. As Simon Sinek's great book suggests, *Start With Why.*

- **Why am I doing this?**
- **Does what I'm doing make sense based on my abilities?**
- **Does this greatly contribute to my primary training goal(s)?**
- **Can I do this? Should I do this? Why or why not?**
- **Is this rational?**

In a fitness industry with a lot of irrationalities and, frankly, insanity about taking workouts to the extreme, we need more rational thinking.

The bottom line is to understand why you do what you do, whether that goes into the **deep science** of building strength or is simply a **common-sense approach** to fitness.

FOCUS ON SAFE STRENGTH

I want to introduce one last key concept to you.

Safe strength is something I feel very strongly about based on my own background as a physical therapist and also overcoming the very serious back injury in my early adulthood.

Here's the specific definition of safe strength.

LIFT AS HEAVY AS POSSIBLE, AS SAFELY AS POSSIBLE, FOR AS LONG AS POSSIBLE.

When is it "too heavy" for safe training?

The load is too heavy when technical failure begins to occur.

It's a point we really don't want to let happen. That's the point where we put the weight down and remind ourselves to lift as heavy as possible but also as safely as possible.

That is how to practice and achieve safe strength.

CHAPTER 12: 8 SIMPLE RULES

"You didn't wake up today to be mediocre."
—T-Nation

In this chapter, I want to share my own rules for training.

These are the key points that underlie my strength training approach and philosophy.

I boiled everything down to just these 8 things.

These rules keep things simple while drilling down to what matters most. It's a set of success standards. If we follow these success standards, we will reap long-term benefits and gain *The Edge of Strength* to keep us moving forward for a long time.

If you're interested in optimizing your health and performance and getting the results you want, then these 8 simple will be a path to get there.

RULE #1: NEVER COMPARE

Never compare yourself to others.

Focus on being the best version of yourself.

If you have the mindset of "Joey's doing better than me" or "Sally can do that and I can't," or whatever it is – that way of thinking is only destructive and self-limiting.

What you need to do is focus on being **YOUR BEST.**

Do not waste your time or energy wallowing about why Joey or Sally is doing better than you.

In life, you will always find that you do better than some in certain situations and there will be others who do better than you. That's the way it is.

If you see someone post a "feat of strength" or some great physical accomplishment on social media, be happy for them, but NEVER compare yourself.

Once again – be YOUR best.

That's all that matters.

RULE #2: OWN YOUR MOVEMENT

We need to move well with basic fundamental movements and also with advanced progressions if we are moving forward in our training.

I've talked about this extensively at this point, so you should know the importance of moving well before moving strong. Chapter 7 also provided examples of how to assess good movement.

By owning your movement, you will work on mastering the basics and also the advanced movement skills that you learn and develop over time.

You will slow down when you need to, take your time with certain exercises, particularly when they are new, and never get careless.

Owning your movement is where it all starts, and from there you can hone your movement skills and gain a deeper understanding what good quality movement is all about.

From the most fundamental exercises such as the deadlift, squat, and press, you should work to perform these movements to your fullest capabilities.

This starts with **keeping good biomechanically efficient techniques.**

And if you have to lower the poundages to do that, your movement quality is something to pay attention to for safe training.

This is owning your movement and being accountable for how well you move during training.

RULE #3: TRAIN INTELLIGENTLY

Listen I love training heavy, but I've learned to train smarter through the years.

We can't afford to do things that hurt our bodies or push ourselves to the brink for extended time periods.

Don't allow yourself to get caught up doing things you know you shouldn't do.

The last chapter talked about being **rational** in our training. We'll also discuss why it's important to focus on the mental aspects of improving ourselves and not just routinely working out.

Training must be a long-term approach.

We can't afford to do careless things like using bad technique, incorporating bad programming, or otherwise beating our bodies into the ground.

Safe training is paramount for short-term and long-term success; that's the bottom-line.

With all the methods and practices I use and teach, there's nothing more important than safety.

On the flip side of that, we can't be so fearful that it stops us from doing anything new, which is also important to train intelligently.

Be sensible and logical about how you approach training.

RULE #4: TRAIN WITH PURPOSE

I've talked about how important it is to know why you train.

Why do you do what you do?

What is your purpose?

What is your one big goal?

Get clear on what you want, put together a plan, and follow the plan through to completion.

Never do things "just because" they look cool or it's the latest shiny new toy in the training arsenal.

This is training with purpose, and **when you have purpose, you have power.**

If you've got a plan, it's like a guided missile towards a result.

> *"Plan the work, and work the plan."*
> *–Dr. Michael Hartle*

There's never a total failure when you execute a plan because the result will be valuable feedback, and that will help you move closer to where you want to be.

If you've got no purpose or plan, it's hard to advance.

Believe me I know because I was stuck at status quo for years until I returned to **training with purpose.**

I got comfortable and got complacent. After getting clear about specific goals and how I could make specific progress in my training, I was able to progress again.

Always have a purpose and a plan, and focus your efforts on the one big thing you've set your sights on.

What do you do when you reach the one big thing and achieve the desired result? Find the next goal, the next target to keep you moving forward down the path to mastery.

I'll talk about the importance of focus in greater detail later when I discuss the 80/20 rule.

For now, remember that you have to know your purpose to get the best results and live to your potential.

Always train with purpose.

RULE #5: RESPECT RECOVERY

Recovery is such a critical factor in the strength training methods advocated in this book. These methods are tough and physically demanding.

Kettlebells, barbell work, and even bodyweight training are all very demanding and taxing on our bodies (depending on many training variables that we are using at a given time).

Recovery methods are critical for:

- optimizing performance
- keeping you injury-free
- avoiding burnout
- making continued progress over the long-term

What kind of recovery method am I talking about? I'm referring to:

- sleep
- stress management and relaxation techniques
- listening to our bodies' cues to rest
- addressing "weak links" through mobilization and flexibility work
- properly restoring and rejuvenating between training sessions and training cycles
- optimizing nutrition and supplementation
- de-loading

Remember, we can't train all out all the time.

This point is often overlooked especially with athletes and "Type A" personalities who want to take their training to the edge.

Type A = high-achieving "train-a-holic"

Managing fatigue, taking time off, taking planned periods of de-loading, meditation, and mobility programs are all ways to manage a healthy state and recover optimally from our training.

We can't forget the importance of using recovery methods strategically in our training approach.

RULE #6: FUEL YOUR MACHINE

I can't stress enough **the importance of great nutrition combined with a high level of training.** We'll discuss this in detail in Chapter 15.

That is the center of a winning combination for health and performance.

Fueling your machine is about getting your body the nutrient-dense foods necessary to perform, recover, and build at a high-level.

Food is fuel for our bodies to perform and function. This is regardless of your age or background. Think of food as high-octane fuel for the machine and the machine is your body.

I'm pretty sure you've heard of the term "garbage in, garbage out," and this is very applicable when talking about feeding your machine. Nutrition is about more than just calories.

Nutrition density is where it at – the vitamins, minerals, and high-quality foods you eat are your fuel.

Again, we'll dive deeper into this very soon in Chapter 15.

RULE #7: FEED YOUR MIND

Always be learning.

Always grow and find ways to improve yourself.

Read books, attend workshops and seminars, listen to podcasts, find mentors, take classes, and put the information into action to advance your knowledge and skill set.

Always be evolving yourself and growing each and every day. This is truly the way to live your strength and discover your greatness.

Once you stop learning and developing, the journey is over, and your potential dies. **Never stop growing and learning.**

> *"When you're green you're growing, and*
> *when you're right you rot."*

That's a mantra to live by.

Seek mastery in the things you do, and try not to jump quickly from interest to interest.

Do or do not; don't dabble.

Masters stay the path while dabblers move from one thing to the next. To read about the master and the dabbler, check out *Mastery* by George Leonard.

The most successful coaches, authors, and entrepreneurs I know are students first. They never stop growing, advancing, and evolving themselves.

If you look at highly successful people you'll find the same thing – they're all active learners and students of life.

Live by **Kaizen,** the principle of constant and never-ending improvement.

RULE #8: HONOR YOUR STRENGTH

You were meant to be strong.

You owe it to yourself to be the strongest version of yourself.

We all have incredible potential to be strong and become the best version of ourselves.

Many simply do not take advantage of that potential.

Honor your privilege to be strong. Don't take it for granted, as most people do.

This book is designed to help you understand the value and benefits of strength, not only in athletic performance but in life performance.

This book offers enough information for people of all levels and backgrounds to choose their strength.

Yes, **strength is a choice.**

As mentioned, there are also many other physical qualities besides strength.

Which ones we focus on depends on the goals or objectives we seek out of our training.

Strength is foundational.

Let's quickly review the 8 rules for long-term strength training.

- RULE #1: NEVER COMPARE
- RULE #2: OWN YOUR MOVEMENT
- RULE #3: TRAIN INTELLIGENTLY
- RULE #4: TRAIN WITH PURPOSE
- RULE #5: RESPECT RECOVERY
- RULE #6: FUEL YOUR MACHINE
- RULE #7: FEED YOUR MIND

- RULE #8: HONOR YOUR STRENGTH

Next, let's talk about 10 specific ways to get stronger.

CHAPTER 13: 10 STRENGTH HACKS

"To get stronger, you need to get stronger."
–Dmity Klokov

A strength hack is a key insight to get you stronger. These are tools, tips, and strategies to improve strength.

First, you need to realize to get stronger, you have to train stronger.

This means train heavier.

You don't get strong using light weights!

Remember what I said earlier about common sense becoming common practice?

STRENGTH IS A SKILL

Strength training is a skill, as you now understand.

We are programming or re-wiring our nervous system to get stronger by practicing the skills of strength, as discussed in Chapter 6.

Strength is primarily the result of the nervous system recruiting more motor neurons.

And, bigger muscles also produce more force. This is how we train and develop the qualities of strength.

Now, let's discuss 10 practical applications to getting stronger – the strength hacks.

MENTAL IMAGERY

You may not have even thought much about this until right now, but why do you think I chose the picture for the cover of this book?

The picture on the cover was selected based on the effective technique of using mental imagery during training.

Mental imagery is powerful and something I've been using for years with great success. When I don't use this technique, the results are less than optimal.

Before you do the lift, see the lift.

For example, when deadlifting, before you do the set, take time to visualize yourself successfully performing the exercise.

Visualize the entire lift and process. See every step and movement in great detail.

- The set-up
- The breathing technique
- The first pull off the ground
- Optimal body mechanics throughout the lift
- The top position – the lock out
- The bar being set back down on the ground
- The exhilaration of you completing the lift

I know it seems very simple, but mental imagery or mental rehearsal is extremely valuable.

Elite athletes use this technique and anyone can learn to use it.

Like anything else, you have to practice the skill of mental imagery.

The more you practice this technique, the greater impact it will have on your outcomes.

JOINT MOBILITY AND MOVEMENT PREP

Always work on joint mobility and movement preparation prior to training, even if only for a few minutes.

Movement preparation is an important part of training. It indirectly helps us get stronger and certainly helps us to train safer.

A simple movement prep program does 3 things to prepare us for training, according to Chad Wesley-Smith of Juggernaut Training Systems.

Benefits of a Movement Prep Program:

- **Increases core temperature**
- **Activates the muscular system**
- **Activates the CNS (Central Nervous System)**

We should work on our movement and mobility skills all the time, even if we already have good movement and mobility.

Otherwise, we tend to lose our muscle flexibility and joint mobility.

Maintaining and improving joint mobility will optimize our training and prevent injury as well.

Work on joint mobility drills and fundamental movement patterns to improve your training.

Have a simple "go-to" movement prep or mobility program that address weak links and fully prepares you for the session ahead.

The goal is always to move better, move with greater strength, and be safe while doing it.

BREATHE

Proper breathing is absolutely essential for strength and power training, yet it's very often missed or underemphasized.

We've covered diaphragmatic breathing in detail in Chapter 7.

Proper breathing will be one of the most valuable techniques you will ever learn.

And as you'll see later, learning **power breathing** with kettlebells is a must.

Similarly, learning how to use the **Valsalva maneuver** for heavy barbells is critical for performance.

Proper breathing makes you stronger, and your lifts will be much safer.

CRUSHING GRIP STRENGTH

Learning how to build your grip strength will enhance your total-body strength.

Pavel Tsatsouline has discussed the importance of grip strength to get stronger.

Grip strength increases full body tension and the ability to produce force. If your grip is weak, your body will be weak. So it's important to have a strong grip to hold barbells, kettlebells, or any heavy object.

Early in my training career, I never realized how important grip strength was to improve overall strength and there's a significant correlation with grip strength and other muscle groups.

One of the great things about grip strength is that it's easy to develop with practice and a high frequency of training.

A great tool to use to radically improve grip strength is **Fat Gripz** for barbells, which increase the circumference of the bar. If you've never used them, you'll be blown away by how taxing they are on the grip with barbell work.

Go to FatGripz.com for more information.

Captains of Crush Hand Gripper is another fantastic way to increase grip strength. These hand grippers are challenging and will develop crushing grip strength. This is something you can keep with you and perform a few reps on a frequent basis.

This technique is known as greasing the groove, where you are practicing a skill frequently at a low level. It works extremely well for training grip strength, and this tool is very effective.

The "Trainer" gripper (100 lb. of resistance) is a good place to start and there are many different levels of resistance to develop grip strength depending on how strong you are.

Go to IronMind.com to learn more.

USE MUSCULAR TENSION

Learning how to use muscular tension during lifts can greatly increase force production making lifts stronger, powerful, and explosive.

Pavel has also taught us the proper use of muscular tension to get stronger.

A specific example of proper use of tension is with the kettlebell military press.

When you press the kettlebell, you are tensing your entire body during the press motion to elevate the kettlebell overhead.

You will find that this gives you much more power to press by using your entire body. That's a way to use tension principles to move with greater strength.

Tension equals strength, but it's also important to recognize the proper balance of tension and relaxation.

For now, simply understand the importance of using tension prior to and during lifts.

We'll cover specifics later when discussing exercises in Section IV.

PROGRAMMING IS KING

On the journey towards better strength, make sure you've got a proper program to get you there.

We'll cover periodization approaches in great detail in Section IV, but know that the most sure-fire path to strength is with a fundamentally solid program.

Lack of focus is easily one of the most self-defeating problems with exercise training. Avoid random training and exercise distractions caused by shiny new toys.

Instead, pick one program and stick to it for the duration.

Failing to plan is planning to fail. A cliché, yes, but it's also the truth.

There are many great strength training programs available. Well-developed programming produces results, and lack of programming produces mediocrity.

PERFORM COMPOUND LIFTS

We need the big lifts to be strong.

Compound lifts involve crossing multiple joints and working many muscles. Examples are:

- **Clean**
- **Clean and press**
- **Deadlift**
- **Squat**
- **Bench Press**
- **Bent Over Rows**
- **Military Press**
- **Snatch**

These multi-joint lifts offer the biggest benefits for pure, raw strength. Big movements produce the biggest strength and have the greatest impact on our bodies.

If you want to include targeted exercises for hypertrophy, make them "accessory" exercises and not the primary focus.

SQUATS AND DEADLIFTS ARE ESSENTIAL

There may be no bigger debate in strength and performance than the following question.

Which is better the squat or the deadlift?

I just mentioned compound, multi-joint movements, which definitely include squats and deadlifts. So they're both excellent exercises.

The truth is you must squat and deadlift (at some level) to fully maximize your strength. If you don't include squats and deadlifts, you're missing out on a lot of potential strength.

Can you get strong without them? Yes.

Will you be stronger with them? Yes.

Learning the proper way to perform these lifts is key, so make sure you spend time with a great strength coach who can show you how to maximize these lifts safely and effectively.

These 2 lifts are fundamental movements for strength, performance, and body composition. They are a critical part of massive functional strength gains.

I'll cover key technical considerations later in the book.

DON'T TRAIN TO FAILURE

There is a misunderstanding about this point.

For the purpose of strength – do not train to failure.

Strength training is extremely taxing on the central nervous system.

It's generally accepted to keep reps in the range of 1 to 5 for strength, but this doesn't mean we take the set to failure.

Taking the heaviest set to failure will fry your nervous system, lead to burnout, and increase the risk of injury.

Deadlifts are extremely physically demanding, and to take a set to failure is a set-up for problems. You want to think about leaving a little gas in the tank, so to speak.

Save your best for competition.

Don't train to failure, at least for strength-training purposes. It's different for hypertrophy because the aim there is muscular failure (which is a totally different process and mechanism).

True strength requires practice, proper technique, sufficient recruitment of muscle fibers, and neuromuscular efficiency, among other things.

This is a key to unlocking strength gains. Train hard, but not to failure. It goes back to the point of strength being a skill.

THE ABS

Strong abs mean a strong body. They're important for total-body stability.

The question is do you have to train the abs specifically to improve total-body strength, or do the abs get stronger as a result of proper training?

I remember reading about a well-known Bulgarian strength coach who scoffed at the idea of doing traditional sit-ups and crunches.

He said that if athletes spent appropriate time doing the big lifts, they would develop far greater benefit with developing abdominal and trunk strength than they could gain by performing sit-ups or crunches.

If we spend more time performing:

- Squats
- Deadlifts
- Barbell (or kettlebell) cleans
- Overhead presses
- All the big lifts advocated in this book

If you'd like to train the abs and trunk stabilizers specifically, one of my favorite things is the ab wheel.

The old-school ten-dollar ab wheel is a fantastic way to develop strong, functional abdominals and superior spinal strength and stability.

No matter what, strong abs mean a stronger body.

SECTION III – PLANNING FOR STRENGTH

"There is only one way to succeed in ANYTHING,
and that is to give it EVERYTHING."
–Vince Lombardi

CHAPTER 14: THE STRONG MIND

"Whether you think you can, or you can't – you're right."
–Henry Ford

As we start to discuss the plan for strength, **everything starts in the mind.**

If we think we can do something, we can usually do it. If we think we can't, we've got no shot.

That's the power of the mind, and quite frankly, mental training doesn't get the attention it deserves in fitness.

The most important thing for success in anything in life is getting your mental game on point.

THE CHAMPION'S MINDSET

If the mind isn't on board with the plan, then how can the body follow?

That's how the wrong mindset can limit growth and sabotage results.

Many people in their 40s and beyond will think that they are too old or past their prime to do exercises that are written in this book.

Well, if that's what they really believe, then that will be "their truth."

"Age is no barrier. It's a limitation you put on your mind."
– Jackie Joyner-Kersee

Again, there are 80-year-olds who compete in Olympic weightlifting and powerlifting.

What do you think their mindset is like?

While many factors contribute to their success, the journey all starts in the mind.

There are many great books about the topic of sports psychology or mindset training. Dr. Jim Afremow wrote *The Champion's Mind*.

When I was able to interview him on **The Rdella Training® Podcast,** he discussed many great concepts around the winning mindset.

However, I want to keep things simple.

Since there's no way to cover a book's worth of information in a chapter, we'll stick to 4 key things that are extremely important for a winning mindset and a strong mind.

These 4 things are the ABCDs of the champions mind.

Keep in mind these are NOT in a particular order, other than the simple alphabetical acronym.

This is to help remember these 4 important components of the strong mind.

A IS FOR ADVERSITY

Every champion and highly successful person learns to deal with adversity.

Since setbacks, challenges, problems, and issues are all part of the process, learning how to deal with and overcome adversity is the key component of a strong mind.

When I went through one of the worst experiences of my life with a major back injury, I knew with certainty that I was going to come back from that injury and compete in bodybuilding again.

That experience changed my life because of my mindset.

And, today I am able to perform at a high training level so many years later.

Overcoming that major challenge taught me so much about handling adversity and having the **mental strength** to endure through tough times.

It taught me about having a vision and being committed to the process.

Expect challenges, expect failures, and expect setbacks because they will happen.

Sooner or later, you will have to learn how to deal with adversity because you never know when hard times will come.

Having the right frame of mind will carry you through those difficulties no matter what challenge you face.

Learning to deal with adversity is a key skill that will make you strong and unstoppable in training and in life.

Embrace adversity, and you will power through life.

Avoid viewing it as the enemy; instead, view it simply as part of the process to make you stronger.

Know that if you endure, you will become stronger.

B IS FOR BELIEF

Belief is critical.

If you don't believe that strength will make you a better person, then this book and the methods that I'm sharing with you will not serve you to the fullest.

You have to believe in the system.

You have to **believe that you are capable of greatness** and that you are capable of closing the gap with your physical potential.

You're capable of a hell of a lot more than you could possibly imagine, and I believe that to be true.

We all have incredible human potential.

Yet the majority simply do not tap into what they have.

Complacency and falling victim to status quo are some explanations, but to be honest, too many people simply don't believe that they can do what's required to get where they want to go.

Let me give you an example.

Many people probably don't believe that they can do Olympic weightlifting for a variety of reasons.

But, they could if they started to believe that they could.

> *"We must do that which we think we cannot."*
> *-Eleanor Roosevelt*

I'm not saying that people can go out and become an Olympic weightlifting champion.

My point is that many more people could engage, at some level, in the skills of Olympic weightlifting.

However, many people would look at the sport as a whole, and their negative self-talk will take over and tell them that they could never do it.

What you can and cannot do starts with belief.

You have to believe in yourself fully.

I'm a big believer in keeping things real. There is a point where belief becomes delusion, and that's not what I'm talking about. I'm talking about a firm belief in yourself and not selling yourself short.

Do you believe in yourself? Do you believe you have the potential for physical greatness?

That is the essence of a champion's mindset.

And, there is no age limit for this, so I don't buy the excuse of I am too old to do this or that. I'm in my late 40s. Again, you have to be real about your abilities, but don't sell yourself short either.

Think big and think bold about what you can do. Ability starts with belief.

C IS FOR CONFIDENCE

"Strong makes life easier.
Strong makes your confidence skyrocket."
–Jen Sinkler

The methods in *The Edge of Strength* will build your confidence more than anything else.

Remember, strength is your edge. The confidence that comes with it will make you unstoppable.

Strengths builds confidence, and confidence builds strength.

Certainly as you get stronger and do more things from a physical standpoint, your confidence and self-esteem will skyrocket to the highest levels.

This shouldn't be surprising.

But, on the other side of that, confidence will build your strength.

As you get more confident with your skills, with your techniques, with your knowledge your strength will go to new levels. And, your results will follow suit.

Your movement, mobility, performance, and body composition will all improve as you get more confident in strength training and the methodologies that are outlined in this book.

Your confidence will make you stronger. However, lack of confidence will limit your strength and forward momentum.

Can you think of any highly successful athletes who aren't confident in what they can do?

LeBron James, Tom Brady, Ronda Rousey, Peyton Manning, Michael Jordan, Serena Williams, or any great champion or athlete that comes to mind.

Do any of these champions lack confidence?

No way.

And, let's not forget the king of confidence – Arnold Schwarzenegger.

No matter what you think about Arnold, I greatly admire his confidence throughout his years as an athlete, actor, entrepreneur, and even politician.

Strength breeds confidence, and if for some reason you lack confidence, strength is a surefire way to skyrocket confidence so it's no longer an issue holding you back.

When you become stronger, you feel more in control. You feel more powerful.

If there is a way to almost instantaneously feel more confident, strength training would be it.

Pick up a heavy loaded bar from the floor, and (as long as your expectations are realistic) you'll feel more confident and powerful immediately after.

Confidence is the key mindset skill and component for a winning life.

D IS FOR DRIVE

This is my favorite component of a winning mindset and a strong mind.

The internal drive I discovered at a young age is why I've been successful in my training and in many things in my life.

If there's one thing that I attribute to the longevity in my training – which includes bouncing back from a major back injury – it's **drive.**

How hungry are you to achieve or excel with your physical self?

The most successful athletes all have this hunger.

Arnold Schwarzenegger, one of the biggest influences in my career, has been so successful because of his intense drive – not only when he was a champion bodybuilder and reigning Mr. Olympia, but with his rise as a movie star and political figure.

Arnold's drive and vision is so admirable.

I've never shared this until now. When I was a young man, I read a quote that radically changed my life. The following statement is from *Arnold, The Education of a Bodybuilder.*

> *"I was relying on ONE thing.*
> *What I had more than anyone else was DRIVE.*
> *I was hungrier than anybody.*
> *I wanted it so badly it hurt.*
> *I knew there could be no one else in the world*
> *who wanted the title as much as I did."*

That, my friend, is drive. This is not to say we all need to be that intense, but this is the ultimate example of a driven mindset.

If you're already driven to excel, then you are way ahead of the game already.

And, if you can find out what really drives you – then you can take things to new levels.

Drive is the internal fire and motivation. It starts with knowing your destination – your reason why you want to be strong.

These keys to the strong mind will help you stop destructive thoughts or emotions like **self-doubt, fear, impatience,** and **negativity** before they get the best of you.

These are the enemies of a winning mindset.

Yet, we've only scratched the surface on mindset. For further reading, check out some of my favorite books on this topic:

- *The Champion's Mind* by Dr. Jim Afremow
- *The Art of Mental Training* by DC Gonzalez

CHAPTER 15: NUTRITION: SIMPLIFIED

"Exercise is king. Nutrition is queen.
Put them together – you have a kingdom."
–Jack LaLanne

How do you know if you're eating right? That depends on how you define good nutrition.

This is a book about strength, but I'd be doing a major disservice to you by not discussing the topic of nutrition.

I'm going to simplify and condense things as best I can to address the link between nutrition and strength.

Nutrition is inherently simple, although this is where most athletes and fitness enthusiasts throw a wrench in their plan. As it's a critical topic, please expand your knowledge further on this subject. Always read and learn more about nutrition for health and peak performance.

One thing you'll find is that there are many different opinions and approaches.

Don't let it overwhelm or confuse you. **Stick to fundamental principles.**

Good nutrition is one of guiding principles in Chapter 12.

Now we'll get into what *fuel your machine* actually means.

If we drill things down to the basics, here are some fundamental principles of nutrition that everyone agrees on:

- **Eat whole, natural foods**
- **Avoid refined, processed grains, sugars, and sugar variants**
- **Eliminate bad fats (trans fats and unhealthy oils)**
- **Don't overconsume**
- **Eat a diet full of nutrient-dense foods**

We also have to remember we are all unique individuals. We all have different genetics, and we have different responses to food.

And, when we're talking about optimizing health, it goes beyond just the food we eat. Optimal health is the interplay of:

- **Exercise**

- **Nutrition**
- **Sleep**
- **Stress Management**
- **Psychological, Emotional and Social Well-being**

While countless nutrition diet plans and books are available, the most effective approaches come back to adhering to good principles of basic nutrition.

THE 4-STEP SYSTEM

This simple system applies whether you're:

- An athlete looking to improve performance
- A recreational exerciser looking to improve body composition
- A fitness enthusiast looking to boost levels of health and energy

STEP 1: WHAT DOES THE SCIENCE SAY?

I am a scientist by nature. That means I look at the scientific evidence and how that relates the human body. When evaluating nutrition, leading with the science is always a good place to start.

Is there some sort of evidence or science behind a theory or rationale?

That's the question I begin with, and we can go to many great books and resources for that information.

For example, does lower carb make sense from a scientific standpoint?

STEP 2: WHAT DOES COMMON SENSE TELL YOU?

Once you look at the scientific evidence, the next step is what does your common sense tell you about the approach?

Does *The Paleo Diet* make sense to you?

Do you understand the basics of it, and does it seem reasonable and sustainable for you?

Depending on your goals and what you like to eat, it might.

Now, what about *The Twinkie Diet?*

Is it reasonable and sustainable?

If no, discard.

If yes, then consider the next step.

STEP 3: TEST THE APPROACH

If there's good science behind a nutritional plan and it makes sense to you, the next step is to test the method.

Ultimately, you have to take action and find out what is going to work best for you. We are all different, and there's only one way to find out how a specific ingredient or dietary plan affects your body.

Try it.

As you test an approach, you have to make sure to give it time. That means you shouldn't try something for a week and claim "that approach didn't work."

You've got to give things a reasonable amount of time to determine the effectiveness. The same thing can be said about training.

STEP 4: FIND OUT WHAT WORKS FOR YOU

Once you start testing different dietary breakdowns or even different foods, you will find out what works best for you.

How long is a reasonable test period to find out what works? Well, 30 days is a good assessment of a nutritional approach or changes to your diet.

If you notice immediate negatives or changes in your body or performance, that's a different story.

In general, shoot for 30 days to assess whether something will work for you or not.

There's a reason behind the method of the WHOLE30® program by Dallas and Melissa Hartwig. Check out Whole30.com for all the details about the program and to get the free PDF of the WHOLE30 Challenge.

Test things out – test foods, test the timing of your meals, test diet plans – and find out what works best for you.

Good nutrition is not complicated, although truly understanding how food interacts with your body can be complex. With that said, we should have a basic understanding of the interactions of the food we eat.

We basically have 3 choices for consuming foods:

- **Proteins**
- **Carbohydrates**
- **Fats**

Everything we eat is composed of a combination of these 3 macronutrients.

We'll talk about macros soon, but how much of each depends on many factors, such as:

- **body type**
- **genetic factors**
- **goals (health, performance, or body composition)**
- **activity levels (sedentary vs. active)**
- **training background**

THINK DIFFERENT

We need to start thinking differently about our nutrition.

It's not just about what you're filling your stomach with right now. We should think about the short-term and long-term benefits or consequences of the food we eat.

The easiest way to think about this is understanding nutrition density. This is the most important principle of good nutrition.

NUTRITION DENSITY IS EATING FOODS THAT ARE RICH, NOT SPARSE, IN NUTRITIONAL VALUE.

Let me give you a specific example.

If you have broccoli or pizza, which one is the more nutrient-dense food?

Broccoli is called a superfood because it's so dense in nutrition. Pizza is not.

Look for whole foods such as:

- **fruits**
- **vegetables**
- **quality lean meats and proteins**
- **healthy fats such olive oil, coconut oil, and avocado**
- **nuts and seeds**

Think of each of these foods in terms of short-term long-term value and benefits.

Let's start with broccoli. If you eat raw broccoli, the short-term benefit is the immediate nutrition density your body gets from the broccoli. The long-term benefit is that your body feels great, you get a high level of nutrients and antioxidants, and it will improve overall health and performance.

Now let's look at pizza. The short-term benefit is the taste. Clearly the majority of people will tell you that pizza is going to taste a lot better than broccoli, right?

But, the short-term consequence is the rapid and significant production of insulin which is not a desirable thing for our body and can lead to insulin resistance if this is done repeatedly over time.

And, **insulin resistance** will lead to other health consequences and even diseases such as Type II Diabetes.

The long-term benefit of eating pizza? Well, there is none.

A typical cheese or pepperoni pizza is not a nutritious food, nor is it healthy for us, especially if consumed excessively and frequently.

Listen, this is not to say you can't eat pizza and I'll be the first to claim pizza as one of my favorite "cheat" foods.

I just make sure that I don't consume it too often. It's a treat or special occasion when I have it – not a standard food in my diet.

What works well for motivating nutritional changes is reframing how you think about foods with this short-term and long-term benefit approach.

I ask myself: does the food I'm eating right now provide short-term and long-term benefits or consequences?

Does it help my body or hurt my body?

Does it add to my health or diminish it in the long run?

Foods that provide maximal nutrition density are always better when judged with this approach.

A BRIEF TALK ABOUT MACROS

Everyone has heard these nutritional terms, but few can explain what they actually mean. Forget the hype about some macros being bad for you because we need all three. Let's review the important roles that macronutrients play in our diet.

PROTEINS

Protein is our building block for muscle tissue and the cells in our body. Our bodies need protein to function optimally, and it is essential for growth.

There are always debates about how much protein we should eat and are high levels of protein necessary. Rest assured that it's extremely difficult to over-consume protein.

If you're training at a high level – and especially for those training for hypertrophy – increased protein consumption would maximize gains and performance.

Without enough protein, how would you expect the muscles to grow, rebuild, and repair?

Another benefit that is well-known is that protein is satiating, which means it helps to satisfy your appetite.

The bottom line is that protein is essential to every strength athlete (that means you), and it's the one macro that remains constant as something to consume more of rather than less.

CARBOHYDRATES

Next up is carbs, which I love to discuss.

Is there a more debated subject in nutrition? Carbohydrates are fuel, but consumed in excess, they are converted to stored body fat.

There's the Paleo approach to reducing carbs, which I do think makes a lot of sense for many people. That's because **most people over-consume the wrong type of carbohydrates.**

But, let's set the record straight: carbohydrate intake depends on many factors, so it's impossible to say what is ideal for you. By no means are all carbohydrates evil.

Here's a quick overview of Paleo:

- **lean, quality proteins, grass-fed beef**
- **fruits and vegetables**
- **nuts, seeds, avocado**
- **olive oil, coconut oil, fish oil**

Yet, we do need carbohydrates to fuel our body. For optimal strength training performance, we just need to focus on consuming the right types of carbohydrates at the right time.

For sedentary people, over-consumption of sugary, processed carbs greatly contribute to overweight and obesity, as well as an overall decline of human health in the world population.

No matter what you do, make sure you're eating the right types of carbohydrates and not over-consuming the bad kind.

Healthy carbs don't come in boxes or packages and have very short ingredient lists, usually consisting of only a single ingredient.

A Paleo approach can work and will be amazing for many people. Keep in mind there are different versions of what Paleo diets should contain. I've been an advocate of the Paleo approach and have followed it myself for many years.

However, I learned that to build muscle, I needed to eat more carbohydrates. Now I'm not carbophobic and I'm certainly not a carboholic.

For building muscle and maximizing hypertrophy, it's nearly impossible to eat a very low-carb diet. When I increase my consumption, I eat more carbs around my training since this is a time when we are more **insulin sensitive.**

We are all different, we are all coming from different training backgrounds, and we have different body types. **There will be many factors determining our carbohydrate intake.**

WHAT YOU NEED TO KNOW ABOUT INSULIN

Insulin is a big deal. It is a hormone secreted by the pancreas to control blood sugar levels.

When we have too much glucose in the blood from carb-heavy meals, it is toxic to the body. That's why insulin is released to help transfer glucose out of the blood as quickly as possible and into body tissues to:

- **be used as fuel**
- **increase glycogen reserves in the muscles and liver, or**
- **be converted into fat and stored in adipose tissue**

When we think about carbohydrates, we must consider insulin response. Every time we ingest carbohydrates, our insulin levels rise to clear blood glucose and store the carbohydrate or glucose into the muscle or liver.

When the muscle and liver has reached its capacity, the remaining glucose must be stored in the body. **It is stored as body fat.** This is the problem with carbs that leads to weight gain and obesity.

If you're training at a high level and your goal is hypertrophy, you have good body composition, and you are already a muscular body type, then you will want to use carbohydrates to replenish the depleted glycogen.

I can't think of any high-level bodybuilder that is following a Paleo type of approach to nutrition. It wouldn't work. They are eating moderate to high level of carbs and doing high-volume hypertrophy training.

Now, the bodybuilder's diet is not necessarily the most optimal way to eat, and things that bodybuilders do to maximize body composition are not always considered "healthy" to be very honest.

But, they are eating for body composition and aesthetics, not optimal health or performance.

To optimize health, we want to maintain insulin levels so that they are not spiking and crashing all the time. In other words, **we want to preserve insulin sensitivity and prevent insulin resistance.**

When eating high carbohydrate and sugary diets, insulin is spiking and crashing repeatedly. At some point insulin will be resistant to the blood sugar spikes, which leads to Type II Diabetes.

We want to eat as healthy as we can; however, we also want to maximize performance in the way that will contribute to our goals.

The amount of carbohydrates to target will vary depending on the individual, the individual goals, and training style and methods.

To enhance lean body mass or reduce body fat, lower carbohydrate consumption will ultimately be necessary. When I followed a low-carb approach for a long time, I lost weight and I actually felt great.

But, with the intense strength training that I do today, it's important to consume more carbohydrates, especially as I'm training for hypertrophy (which we should always be doing).

I've personally asked some of the top nutrition experts, Paleo authorities, and thought leaders this question...

"Can you build muscle on a low-carb diet?"

The answer is no, you cannot. At least not when paired with the type of heavy training discussed in this book.

Muscles need carbohydrates and store them as glycogen in the muscle (also stored in the liver). The thing is, our bodies only hold so much glycogen (~500 grams) in the skeletal muscle and liver.

After that, the glucose (carbohydrate) is converted to – you guessed it – fat.

If shedding stored fat is one of your primary goals, Abel James in his book *The Wild Diet* summarized the **secret to fat loss** in just one sentence – **stay away from sugar and processed grains, especially in the morning.**

A CRASH COURSE IN FATS

All fats are not equal. The major types of fats to be concerned with are:

- **Saturated fats**
- **Monounsaturated fats (MUFAs) Omega 3s**
- **Polyunsaturated fats (PUFAs) Omega 6s**
- **Trans Fatty Acids (TFAs) and partially-hydrogenated oils**

Except for TFA and the partially-hydrogenated oils, fats are critical for metabolic function and general health.

It still surprises me that some people believe fat is the enemy. What we want to avoid are the unhealthy trans fats and partially-hydrogenated oils.

Examples of unhealthy trans fats include:

- processed, packaged junk foods and frozen foods
- vegetable oils (including canola oil) and seed oils
- margarine

- baked and packed goods

We also want to have a good ratio of the omega 6 to omega 3 fats (approximately 2:1 or even 1:1 – omega 6 to omega 3).

A typical diet can contain a very high ratio of omega 6 to omega 3 fatty acids, so we want to narrow the gap in the ratio to promote health and reduce systemic inflammation.

Healthy fats include:

- Grass-fed, organic, and/or pastured animal fats like butter, meats, eggs
- Wild-caught fish that are high in omega 3s
- Avocado
- Olive oils
- Coconut Oil

One final thing to keep in mind. **If you increase fat intake, carb intake should be reduced and vice versa.**

Remember what I said about **protein being the constant macronutrient?**

FOOD QUALITY

The training philosophy I've been telling you about means nothing without great nutrition.

For both health and performance, we need the highest quality of foods to fuel our bodies. Nutrition is the major limiting factor that prevents people from achieving the things they want.

Do most of your foods come in packages and boxes? Or are they whole, natural, fresh foods?

Great nutrition is a result of habits.

Remember the laws from Chapter 8? First was the law of individual differences. Here's a great example of how we're different.

Why does caffeine affect certain people more than others? Some people get anxious and jittery if they consume too much coffee (or caffeine) while others aren't affected much at all.

Some people have a specific enzyme in the liver that breaks down caffeine much more rapidly than others. Because of this, they don't experience the over-stimulation effects because caffeine is cleared more rapidly. When others have less of this enzyme, caffeine is broken down much more slowly, and as a result they feel the effects of caffeine to a much greater extent.

This is the law of individual differences, or more specifically, genetic polymorphism.

Genetic polymorphism is defined as the differences in genetic make-up between individuals.

We're different, yet we're all the same.

While we do have genetic differences between us, all humans are working with the same basic biological systems. There are certain basic fundamental principles for good nutrition that we can all follow.

There are so many "diets" and nutritional approaches, it gets overwhelming. As with my approach to training, I'm a big believer in keeping things simple. When all is said and done, there are 2 major problems I typically see with regards to nutrition.

- **Lack of understanding**
- **Poor habits**

The solution is simply to better understand food's interaction with our body and develop the right habits. We'll discuss habits soon.

For one of the best books on habit development pertaining to nutrition and exercise, I highly recommend checking out *Fat Loss Happens on Monday* by Josh Hillis and Dan John.

DIETS

There's the Paleo Diet, the Slow Carb Diet, the Velocity Diet, the Zone Diet, the Mediterranean Diet, the Bulletproof Diet, the Wild Diet, and even the Badass Diet (yes, I'm serious).

You get the point.

There's no single "right" diet for all people. How we plan to eat is largely dependent on what our goals are.

For example, if hypertrophy is the primary goal and you're training with high intensity and volume with resistance exercise, it's going to near-impossible to put on size with a lower carb approach, as I mentioned.

But, for Joe – the couch potato – who wants to lose 20 pounds of excess body fat, a paleo-type approach is probably going to be magical.

SIMPLE PRINCIPLES

Let me cut to the chase and cover some key considerations that are universal for all of us, regardless of goals. These are basic nutritional habits for optimal health.

FOCUS ON NUTRIENT-DENSE FOODS

This is pretty obvious, but we want to eat foods that are nutritionally dense. If you did this one thing, it would guarantee improved health.

A great way to think about nutrient-dense foods (or whole foods) are foods that have only one ingredient.

Vegetables are key. You can never eat enough vegetables and they are the ultimate in nutritional density, so load up. One recommended nutritional practice for all humans is to eat an abundance of vegetables.

Foods that are packaged or processed are rarely loaded with the nutrients you need to fuel your body. This is what we want to avoid or reduce.

We especially want to avoid or minimize the refined grains, sugars, and highly processed oils (such as vegetable oils). These are problematic for health, performance, and for body composition. And, they serve little to no nutritional purpose.

EAT MORE PROTEIN

As discussed in the section about macros, **protein is the constant.** It's essential for health and muscle tissue and repair.

The general rule for most people, especially those who follow *The Edge of Strength* training approach, is **.7 to 1 gram of protein per pound of bodyweight.**

You may find different recommendations, depending on who or where you read, but in my conversations with nutrition experts, this is the recommendation I've heard the most.

This simple way to eat more protein is to ensure you have a fist-size portion with every meal. Build all your meals around protein, and you'll always have enough to fuel your strength and recovery.

DRINK MORE WATER

Our bodies are approximately 70% water.

Drinking water is critical to our health and performance.

Most don't drink enough or they drink the wrong kinds of beverages (soda, sugary drinks, even alcohol). **A general rule of thumb is to drink a half ounce of water per pound of bodyweight.**

Here's a quick test to see if you're hydrated. If your urine is pale and colorless, you're probably getting enough water, but if it's yellow or dark, you need more fluid.

USE NUTRIENT TIMING (NT)

NT is simply using the right nutrients at the right time, basically around your training.

NUTRIENT TIMING (NT) IS THE STRATEGIC MANIPULATION OF NUTRITION, TO ENSURE THE GREATEST BENEFIT FROM EXERCISE AND PEAK PERFORMANCE.

In combination with the training methods I cover in this book, I have been an advocate of using the principles of nutrient timing (NT) for a long time.

The way that I most commonly NT is to use approximately 20–30 grams of a carbs and proteins in combination pre – and post-training. The ratios don't seem to matter so much. Just make sure you consume a combination of carbohydrate and protein.

There are several benefits of this:

- **Increase nutrient delivery to the muscles**
- **Minimize muscle damage**
- **Promote recovery benefits**
- **Shift metabolism to anabolic state**
- **Take advantage of insulin sensitivity**
- **Promote muscle protein synthesis**

The discussion on NT can be extensive, so I recommend checking out books and research articles written on the subject. Although *Nutrient Timing* by John Ivy and Robert Portman is a bit dated, it's still one of the best resources to learn about the benefits of nutrient timing.

While the research seems to change each year, common sense says that it's an effective strategy to use to optimize training performance and recovery.

GOOD NUTRITION IS ABOUT HABIT BUILDING

What you eat will always depend on your habits – planning, preparing, cooking, packing, shopping, etc.

Eat the right foods, and eat them frequently. That's just part of what you can do to support better health every day. We learn, we apply, and we see what works for each us.

Good nutrition is an eating pattern that provides you ideal health, body composition, and performance.

And, that's just the truth.

Once again, body type, training goals, genetics, and training methods ALL play a huge factor in optimizing nutrition.

EATING STRATEGY "CHEAT SHEET"

Here's the ultimate guide to helping you eat for different goals.

WEIGHT LOSS

QUANTITY (I.E., CALORIC DEFICIT)

While I'm not a fan of **calorie counting** in general, caloric deficits (eating less than what your body expends) is effective and obviously makes sense for weight loss.

There are problems with this, including the rebound effect.

Intermittent fasting (IF) may be a viable option and has received much attention for health and weight loss benefits. There's many ways to use IF, so research the subject more to find out if it may be an option for you.

No matter what, resistance training must be a part of the weight-loss equation.

FAT LOSS

FOOD QUALITY & MACRONUTRIENT RATIOS

For fat loss, a reduction or manipulation of carbs will be beneficial with an increase in fat intake. You must reduce or eliminate sugar.

Manipulation of macronutrients is a key to fat loss, I learned that many years ago as a competitive bodybuilder.

BUILDING MUSCLE

CARBS – THE RIGHT ONES

To build muscle you need to consume adequate carbs and protein. Reference the carbohydrates section of this chapter for more information on this.

For a reasonable and well-explained position on carbohydrate intake, read Nate Miyaki's *The Truth about Carbs*.

ATHLETIC PERFORMANCE

NUTRIENT TIMING

Fueling for optimal performance and recovery is about when you consume what nutrients. This means using appropriate foods pre- and post-training, as we've covered.

SUPPLEMENTATION

I hate to see exaggerated claims about weight loss, muscle building, and performance supplements.

Why would we need to take supplements if we're eating with maximal nutrition density? Supplements are supplemental. We shouldn't depend on them, but they can definitely help when training at a high level.

With this in mind, the supplements below are the proven winners based on my experience and according to the scientific evidence. They can offer convenient ways to get the right nutrient timing.

PROTEIN SUPPLEMENTS

Protein supplements are a way to meet daily protein requirements. Protein is satiating and is the essential build block for muscle growth.

Since protein is the "constant" macronutrient, you'll want to make sure there's a steady supply of it in your diet.

The key with protein supplements (powders or bars) is to make sure they are high-quality protein, minimally processed, and low in sugars and fillers.

Here's my checklist for protein powders:

- **Grass-fed Whey is preferred (although I have found some great plant-based proteins)**
- **Minimal ingredients – the shorter the list, the better**
- **As 'clean' as possible – long chemical names are a no-go**
- **No sugar (or sugar alternatives) except a low amount of stevia**

FISH OIL

When you're training at a high level, there are a few supplements I would definitely recommend for optimal health and recovery. Fish oil is one of them. Not just any fish oil, but a **high-quality fish oil.** All fish oils are not created the same.

There's a large body of research about the health benefits of fish oil. Omega-3 fatty acids are important for immune function and for decreasing inflammation.

The EPA and DHA fatty acids found in fish oils are famous for promoting numerous health benefits that aid in preventing many major life-threatening diseases.

After exercising, your immune system becomes suppressed, and systemic inflammation can occur, especially with high-intensity resistance training.

To help counteract this immune system stress and inflammation, take quality fish oil that contains healthy omega 3s with generous doses of EPA and DHA. These are beneficial for your body in terms of health and recovery.

CREATINE MONOHYDRATE

Creatine is the most studied sports nutritional supplement on the market. The benefits of creatine are both impressive and compelling for performance, aesthetics, and overall health.

While creatine is extremely effective, the reports on creatine usage are sometimes inaccurate and misleading.

Creatine is a naturally occurring amino acid-like compound, found primarily in skeletal muscle (about 95% of creatine is in the muscle). The body typically stores around 120 grams of creatine at any given time, but does have the capacity to store even more, up to 160 grams.

Your body can replenish creatine either by diet, with foods that contain creatine such as beef and salmon or you get creatine from the synthesis from the amino acids, glycine, arginine, and methionine.

Numerous studies have shown that dietary supplementation of creatine monohydrate **increases the creatine muscle stores by 10-40%.**

Supplementing allows creatine storage in the body to be at full capacity, rather than at 75% of its capacity.

Data has suggested that higher levels of muscle creatine correlate well with **increased performance,** specifically in short bouts of exercise training requiring creatine as energy, such as weight training or sprinting.

Creatine supplementation **primarily benefits strength/power athletes** or anyone looking to increase strength, increase lean muscle mass, and improve athletic and/or training performance.

What about the side effects?

There is only one clinically significant side effect that has been reported in over 1000 studies to date. That side effect is weight gain, which is typically due to an increase in muscle mass, as opposed to fluid retention.

Research has shown that a short period of loading is the best way to rapidly increase creatine stores in the muscle. A typical loading/dosing regimen would include loading for 5-7 days at a dose of 15-25 grams, then taking **3-5 grams per day to maintain.**

Creatine has been shown to increase exercise work output, increase strength performance, and increase muscle mass.

Research has shown that it's safe and effective, both in the short term and with long-term usage.

VITAMIN D

Vitamin D is recognized today as a critical supplement for health and performance. And, it's been reported that high numbers of people are either **deficient or insufficient** in Vitamin D (insufficient is much more severe).

Vitamin D is a low-cost supplement that offers many benefits for health and performance, especially when training at high levels. Benefits include:

- **Increased bone health**
- **Boosts the immune system**
- **Improved muscle function**
- **Improved performance**
- **Low levels correlate to a number of serious diseases**

There's really no reason not to take Vitamin D as insurance when you consider all the upsides of such an inexpensive and valuable supplement.

Dosing will vary. I typically take 2500 IUs per day.

GREENS

Another insurance policy for optimal health is a good greens supplement. A glass of greens is a glass full of dense nutrients.

I'm a big fan of greens supplements for the simple reason that it's extremely hard to over-consume greens. If you take a single serving of a good greens product, it ensures that you're getting in your daily dose of complete nutritional density.

First thing in the morning in a fasted state, I like to take my greens to load the body with high nutrition upon waking. When I do this, it tends to start the day out great, and I feel physically and psychologically fantastic.

There is one problem with greens, though.

Frankly, the taste with many products is bad.

There are brands that actually taste decent, so I'd encourage you to taste test a few to see which ones will work for you.

These are my primary supplements. Others I utilize include **magnesium, caffeine,** and some "clean" **pre-workout products** that I've discovered.

CHAPTER 16: STRONG HABITS

*"Small disciplines, repeated with consistency every day,
lead to great achievements gained slowly over time."*
–John C. Maxwell

Our habits make us stronger.

We are creatures of our habits, and habits greatly impact strength and performance.

This book is about maximizing human potential and performance. In order to do that, we need the right habits. If we get married to a bad routine, we'll be stuck in the status quo. **With the right habits, we can achieve peak performance and excellent results.**

Our habits make us who we are.

In this chapter, I want to share some key habits that will make a difference in optimizing your health and performance. These are simple things that anyone can do to improve themselves.

And, I've got a simple and effective **3-step process** for long-term habit development.

I'm always working on my own habits because they are the secret to improving our lives. Let's just take the habit of reading, for example. This is something I'm extremely passionate about.

Daily reading is something so simple and can dramatically improve your knowledge, brain power, and the quality of your life in almost every way. Yet, many people prefer to plop down on the couch and flip on the TV for hours at a time.

It's a lot easier to be a couch potato. You don't have to think or doing anything. It's completely mindless and passive.

If that's how you're spending your time, it's a result of having the wrong habit. But, it's actually easy to fix.

GREAT HABITS LEAD TO SUCCESS

Whether you're a general fitness enthusiast or a high-level competitive athlete, you can improve your habits to make you even better.

Where you are right now is a direct result of your daily habits. Likewise, **the person you want to become is a by-product of your daily habits.**

You and I probably have different habits we want to develop.

For many people, developing new, powerful habits can range from something as simple as drinking more water or eating more vegetables, to more challenging goals like training 5 days per week or practicing meditation daily.

The right habits change lives.

The more I learn about the power of habits, the more I'm convinced that this is truly what defines our success.

Wrong habits can prevent us from being what we're capable of becoming.

Life-changing habits can be related to:

- **eating**
- **training and recovery**
- **sleeping**
- **managing stress**
- **self-improvement**

As I write this, I know there are habits I need to develop to evolve myself to the level I want to be.

What about you?

If we take one habit at a time, one baby step at time a time, that will lead to long-term success.

The little things add up over time.

Leo Babauta in his great book *The Power of Less* discussed the importance of having only one goal per month.

He reported an 80% success rate with people who followed the one goal per month rule.

For those who attempt 2 or more goals, the success rate dips to below 20%!

If you're serious about developing habits, tackling one per month is the way to go.

The key to developing great habits comes down to focusing on a few things.

According to Charles Duhigg in his great book, *The Power of Habit*, there are 3 major stages of habit development. Duhigg's "habit loop" contains the cue, the routine, and the reward.

Here's how this works, outlined using a specific example of how I've applied it to increase daily water consumption.

THE CUE

As I set out to consume more water each day, my cue was an empty glass I would leave out on the counter.

When I woke up and headed for the kitchen in the morning, I would see the empty glass (the cue).

It immediately would remind me to fill it and drink a full glass of water first thing in the morning.

THE ROUTINE

As I continued to do this every day, it became more routine to put out the glass.

Then I saw the glass, I filled it, drank it, and that's it.

The simple cue led to the routine.

THE REWARD

Ultimately, there has to be a reward for the routine to become conditioned as a habit.

The reward is that I immediately feel better when I drink water. I know my body needs water, especially in the morning when I wake from an overnight fast.

The immediate feeling I get after a glass of water is rewarding because I feel better, just from rehydrating my body.

The reward doesn't seem like much, but it's noticeable.

Habits should become automatic and effortless. When these 3 steps align, it's the root of habit development.

CUE + ROUTINE + REWARD = HABIT

What if we established one new habit a month for a year?

In a year, we would have 12 new, powerful habits and that would make a huge difference, don't you think?

STRENGTH HABITS

Let's look at 10 powerful habits related to training success and personal development that can make a big difference.

These are habits for the strength athlete (that would be you).

HABIT #1: HAVE A MORNING RITUAL

A morning ritual is a key habit, series of habits, or routine that you do first thing in the morning.

It sets up your day for total success.

This can be as simple as drinking a glass of water. Or it can be much more comprehensive with things like:

- Nutritious breakfast
- Reading
- Planning the day
- Stretching
- Mediation
- Writing or journaling
- Training session/workout

I've discovered in recent years that successful people and athletes have these morning rituals, or success rituals, and everyone does them a little different.

My morning ritual changes from time to time, but I typically always do something like this:

- A simple dental health routine (see habit #4)
- Drink a full glass of water upon rising
- Eat a nutrient-dense meal
- At least 10 minutes to read
- 10 minutes to "fine tune" the day's agenda

To learn all about morning rituals, check out *The Morning Miracle* by Hal Elrod.

HABIT #2: DRINK MORE WATER

This habit is so simple but just as easily overlooked.

Drinking water is critically important for health and performance. Hopefully we agree on that.

Yet, many of us don't drink enough water.

Many of us are in fact chronically dehydrated.

We discussed how much water you should drink in the last chapter, and it's important enough to go over again here.

According to the book *Your Body's Many Cries for Water*, a general rule of thumb is to **drink a half ounce of water per pound of bodyweight.**

For a 200 pound individual, they would drink 100 ounces of water per day. That's over 12 cups of water, the equivalent of about 8 cans of soda – but do not drink soda.

HABIT #3: DELIBERATE PRACTICE

Do you approach your training with the intent of getting a little bit better each session?

We discussed in Chapter 6 – Strength Science, how practice builds myelin in the nervous system, which leads to better skill and performance.

Practice isn't just an action. It's a habit.

Don't just workout by performing a gym routine. Practice and refine your skills, especially with the methods and techniques I'll share with you soon in this book.

Apply the 1% rule to make little improvements every day.

Practice doesn't make perfect; practice makes permanent.

Make sure you practice right.

HABIT #4: TAKE CARE OF YOUR TEETH

This habit probably sounds funny, I know, but dental health is intimately related to overall health.

The work by Weston Price, specifically the book *Nutrition and Physical Degeneration,* covers the important relationship between nutrition, health, and your teeth.

Take care of your teeth, and that includes flossing every day.

Flossing, in particular, has been linked to the incidence of heart disease.

Leave the floss out as a cue to build this habit if you don't have it already.

HABIT #5: PLAN YOUR MEALS

There is no doubt that meal planning is a critical habit.

The better I plan, the easier it is to eat well, and the more successful my nutrition is.

Here's what happens when you don't plan. You eat on the run and usually end up eating low-nutrient foods.

But, when you plan ahead and prepare your meals or snacks, the calm, rational you is in control. Therefore, you are in a position to set yourself up for success.

Meal planning can include physically cooking and preparing your meals ahead of time.

Or, planning could be knowing where you're going to get your major meals from so that you aren't eating on the fly.

When I pack my lunch, do you know what I do? I leave the food container out on the counter as a reminder (the cue).

Meal planning is a key habit for all us.

HABIT #6: PROTEIN AT EVERY MEAL

If protein is the constant macro, as I've mentioned, then we need to eat protein at every meal.

How much?

A great guideline I've seen is a fist-size portion of protein.

Your fist is with you everywhere you go, right? It's a quick measure of how much protein to eat with each meal.

HABIT #7: EAT VEGETABLES 3X DAILY

I can't think of anyone I know (myself included) who wouldn't benefit from eating more vegetables.

You can consume vegetables in unlimited quantity.

Have you ever heard of anyone getting fat, out of shape, having health issues, or feeling bad by over-consuming vegetables? Me either.

Green leafy vegetables and colorful vegetables should be consumed in abundance. This is something that all thought leaders and nutrition experts agree on.

The easy way to develop a habit of consuming vegetables is to eat them every day.

Once you've got that down, try to eat vegetables a minimum of three times a day – with lunch, dinner, and as a snack or supplement (using a greens product counts as a serving).

HABIT #8: READ DAILY

"You dropped 150 grand on an education that you could've got for $1.50
in late charges at the public library."
–Good Will Hunting

I'm a voracious reader. Of course I've learned many of the lessons that constitute *The Edge of Strength* by training myself, but many insights can also be attributed to the habit of reading.

Reading is a powerful way to develop yourself, and strong people are those who continue to develop themselves. Yes, this book is about physical strength, but really it's about discovering the best version of yourself.

If I can give you one big piece of advice to practice the 1% rule, **you have to read every day.** Whether you actually read or listen to audio, make it part of your daily success routine or ritual.

You're reading this book, so I assume you are a reader.

I encourage you to read more, learn more, and devour great books. Then put things into action.

Too busy to read?

Try reading for just 10 minutes each day.

Reading will make you better in almost every way and it's so easy to do.

You sit down, open up a book, and go.

No matter how busy we are, we all have at least 10 minutes to do this.

And, what happens is that we usually end of reading for much longer.

Make 10 minutes of reading a day a habit, and you'll end up reading beyond an hour a week.

What if you read a book a month?

That's 12 new books a year.

What if you read a book a week?

That's 52 books a year and a **"world-class education."**

HABIT #9: MANAGE STRESS

Chronic stress is a health and performance killer. From a body composition standpoint, elevated cortisol can wreak havoc.

Interested in why? I highly recommend reading *Why Zebras Don't Get Ulcers* by Robert Sapolsky to learn more about the science of chronic stress.

Stress management is one of those under-the-radar topics that gets lost when we're talking about strength and performance. Yet, it can be the difference to getting great results and average results.

How do you recognize stress, let alone manage it? Here are some simple habits to build for stress management:

- Deep breathing techniques
- Meditation
- Short naps
- Relaxation methods

- Consistent sleep patterns
- Massage
- Outdoor walks
- Foods that keep you in hormonal balance
- A 10-minute movement and mobility program
- Daily reading or writing

We must find ways to manage our stress to optimize our health and performance.

Ten minutes a day of stress management can be all it takes. All you have to do is find a method that works for you.

HABIT #10: PRACTICE GRATITUDE

This habit is simple.

Be grateful for what you've got.

Practice being grateful every day.

Be grateful for where you are and what you have.

Don't take it for granted.

I've found many successful people who take a few minutes at the end of the day to write down the top 3 things they're grateful for.

It's only a few minutes, but it gives you perspective and appreciation. It gives you time to reflect on how you've grown in the short – and long-term.

The daily practice of gratitude can be a life changer, and that's why I wanted to share it here.

DEVELOPING NEW HABITS

So, how long does it take to develop a new habit?

Well, that all depends on what you read.

There is evidence that it takes as long as 66 days, but most of what you'll find is that it takes about 30 days.

In general, I do think that 30 days is about right for most people. It's at least a good amount of time to try out something new and then assess how it's affecting your life.

Habits are powerful, and our habits shape us.

Our habits make us stronger.

Let's recap the 10 simple power habits:

1. Have a Morning Ritual
2. Drink More Water
3. Deliberate Practice
4. Take Care of Your Teeth
5. Plan Your Meals
6. Protein at Every Meal
7. Eat Vegetables 3 Times a Day
8. Read Daily
9. Manage Stress
10. Practice Gratitude

What are a few habits you can start to work on right now that will contribute to your big goals?

List habits to work on below:

_____

_____

_____

_____

_____

_____

_____

_____

CHAPTER 17: FINDING PURPOSE

"Clarity is Power."
–Tony Robbins

I've given the WHY. Now, we get to the WHAT.

Specifically, what is it you want to get out of your training?

When you have clarity regarding your goals, you've won half the battle already. A major stumbling block for people is lack of purpose.

Lack of clarity.

This chapter solves that problem. Let's look at how to overcome one of the biggest challenges in 5 simple steps.

THE ONE THING

As the cliché goes, if you don't know where you're going, any road will get you there.

Narrowing down **one goal at a time** is how you get perpetual results for the rest of your life. This is how you move out of the status quo and go from **ordinary to extraordinary.**

First, let's talk about what getting clear is not. "Getting in better shape" is not a clear goal. It doesn't mean anything unless it's objective and measurable.

The following examples are clear because they're quantifiable.

BODY COMPOSITION:

- Achieve or maintain 10% body fat
- Reduce belly fat circumference by 1"
- Losing 10 pounds (while it's objective, it's not always a good goal because, if you add quality muscle while reducing fat, the weight may not really matter)
- Fitting comfortably into your favorite jeans or clothes (your clothes don't lie, making it a great objective measure for progress)

FITNESS/PERFORMANCE:

- Deadlifting 2x bodyweight

- Pressing a 40 kg kettlebell
- Competing in your 1st PL meet (competition is a phenomenal goal, a great way to get laser focused, and also a great way to get out of your comfort zone)
- Being able to successfully perform a bodyweight barbell snatch with solid technique
- Standing long-jump improvement (pre/post training program)

AESTHETIC/VISUAL:

- Get before and after pictures when completing a program
- Measure body part circumferences (e.g., arms, chest, legs) before and after hypertrophy based programs
- Use the mirror (the simple way to assess progress for aesthetic goals)

ROUTINE/ENERGY:

- Having sustained energy without mid-afternoon crashes
- Sleeping 8 hours each night with interrupted sleep (going to bed and rising at same time each day)
- Using specific pre and post workout nutrition for each training session
- Develop a structured morning routine or success ritual each and every day (you either have it or you don't, you either do it or you don't)

We can measure any of these. Specificity is the key. That's why progress seems easier for high-level athletes. They know EXACTLY what they want.

Well, you can too.

5 STEPS TO GETTING WHAT YOU WANT

We all basically have 3 major goals:

- **Performance** – The do-better goal
- **Aesthetics** – The look-better goal
- **Health** – The feel-better goal

Motivation is whatever gets you going.

And, what gets us going can be boiled down to 2 things:

- Pain / loss (move away from)
- Pleasure / victory (move towards)

Some of us are much more motivated by pleasure than pain and vice versa. Understanding your motivation gives you leverage to succeed.

Now, I have an exercise for you.

I want to highly encourage you to do the exercise below. Whether you're a novice or approaching Level 5 strength, gaining clarity on your training goals is always valuable to do.

It's time to re-focus.

This is great to do every few months, maybe once per quarter, as things change, and we should always re-assess where we are and what we want.

GETTING CLEAR

You can do this exercise in the book or take out a blank piece of paper – the main thing is to do this right now.

STEP 1: MAKE A LIST

Make a list of the top 10 health and/or fitness goals you'd like to work on and achieve in the next 3–6 months.

Think about specific outcomes, something objective and measurable, and a goal that is actionable and achievable.

List 10 things here – I'm pretty sure we can all come up with 10 things we'd like to achieve.

_____

_____

_____

_____

_____

_____

_____

STEP 2: FIND THE ONE THAT'S MOST IMPORTANT

Out of those 10 things, circle the #1 MOST important goal to your right now.

THIS IS YOUR FOCUS.

Congratulations, you just got clear on what you want!

> *"When you know what you want,*
> *and you want it bad enough,*
> *you will find a way to GET IT."*
> *– Jim Rohn*

Next, we have another important step with this.

STEP 3: KNOW WHY

What makes the goal you circled most important to you right now?

WHY is this a must for you, and WHY now?

Having a strong why gives you massive leverage, as we've discussed. If you don't have a strong enough reason WHY, it's not likely you'll achieve the goal – that's the harsh truth.

The stronger the reason you have to do something, the more likely you will be to achieve it. When you have to work towards your goal but have low energy and motivation, it makes it tough. Your "why" has to compel you into action.

This is a very important step.

STEP 4: IDENTIFY OTHER IMPORTANT GOALS

Next, put a star or check by 2 to 3 more items on that list that are in alignment or could complement the primary goal.

Here's an example.

Let's just say you have a performance goal. You want to deadlift 400 pounds (or whatever that number is for you).

Maybe there are 2 or 3 things on the list that could be accomplished as a by-product of focusing on that top goal.

Examples:

- Gain 5 pounds of quality muscle (Yes)
- Complete a 6-week or 12-week structured program (Yes)
- Press half bodyweight with a kettlebell (Yes)

Now you've accomplished more of your goals by **focusing on your one thing.**

Remember that goals must be congruent with each other and not opposing. You can't expect to achieve max deadlift and train for your 1st ironman event at the same time – that doesn't work.

To prioritize in one area is to de-prioritize in another area.

But, you may find other things on that list that can be accomplished by focusing on the primary goal, providing they are related to one another. Have a few clearly defined things you want to achieve, but keep your eye on the one big thing.

For more on this approach, I highly recommend the phenomenal book *The One Thing* by Gary Keller and Jay Papasan. The book is one I constantly recommend to others and refer back to with many life-changing concepts.

STEP 5: IDENTIFY WHAT YOU MUST DO

What do you need to do, specifically, to achieve your ONE BIG thing? Here are some examples:

- Program – what program matches the goal?
- Skills – what new skills or techniques do you need to develop?
- New Habits – what new habits do you need?
- Coaching – who can help you?
- Live workshop or course – is there are course or seminar you can take to accelerate your progress?
- Research – what book or books do you need to read?
- Nutrition – what nutrition changes do you need to make?
- Consistency – how will you ensure consistency to meet this goal?
- Tools/equipment – do you need any new tools or equipment?
- Stress management – how will you manage stress, sleep, and recovery?
- Support system – what additional support do you need?

What are the key things you need that will enable to achieve this goal? List them out, whatever they are.

Take the time to do this simple exercise. And then keep the information in front of you at all times.

Keep the goal on your desk, hang it somewhere you can see it, and do what it takes to keep it relevant.

Finally, get to work.

THINKING LONG-TERM

No matter what you think about goal-setting, the fact is we need something to drive us forward. We need to be clear, focused, and driven towards one big thing at all times.

Yet, what we want may not be what we need.

For example, you may want to look and feel better (of course we'd need to be much more clear on what that really means). But, what you need is a solid strength-training program and overhaul of your nutrition fundamentals.

That doesn't mean you shouldn't set your sights high.

What successful person doesn't dream big and bold about what can be accomplished?

B.H.A.G. – THE BIG HAIRY AUDACIOUS GOAL

An idea conceptualized in the book *Built to Last* by Jim Collins that described the long-term vision of successful companies.

We can repurpose this from the business world for the purposes of strength-training.

The B.H.A.G. goal is the #1 goal (the REALLY big goal) you'd like to achieve if you think as big and bold as you can.

THINK OF THE ONE BIG, BOLD GOAL THAT EXCEEDS WHAT YOU THINK IS POSSIBLE.

For a specific strength goal, it's easy to see how this work.

You could have a B.H.A.G. for a specific deadlift number, whether that's 400 pounds or 800 pounds.

This really big goal gives us purpose, passion, hope, excitement, and vision.

It keeps us thinking big about what we can accomplish if we keep going long-term.

If we don't achieve the B.H.A.G., we don't need to be disappointed or feel defeated. It's about the journey and the process to keep us moving forward.

Go down the right path, and the results will follow.

I remember a conversation with top strength coach Josh Bryant, who said, "There is no such thing as failure, there is only a result."

THE ONE-GOAL SYSTEM

Here's some more examples of B.H.A.G.

Remember, we are all different and coming from different backgrounds. These are just examples to illustrate the point:

- Deadlift 500 pounds
- Squat 400 pounds
- Barbell Snatch bodyweight with safe technique
- Press 1/2 bodyweight with a kettlebell
- Perform a kettlebell bent press with 36 kg kettlebell
- Successfully complete a kettlebell snatch test
- Perform 10 strict tactical pull ups
- Perform a pistol squat
- Complete 500 kettlebell swings in one training session
- Compete in your 1st weightlifting meet
- Win your next competition

This is also how I approach **Strength Stacking,** which we'll discuss in Chapter 19.

Be clear and consider having a B.H.A.G. to keep you thinking big and bold about your long-term potential.

Having one big goal at a time is amazing and effective.

It's made a huge difference for me, and I know it can work for you too, especially if you use the five-step method to get clear on what you want out of your strength training.

Find your B.H.A.G., and get to work on it. Let it drive your success.

CHAPTER 18: THE POWER OF 80/20

"The elite are the elite because they are better
at the fundamentals than everyone else."
–Unknown

This is an intentionally short chapter for a reason. It's about FOCUS.

The Edge of Strength System is simple. It's about focusing on the fundamentals or what's most important.

This is also known as the 80/20 rule:

80% OF YOUR RESULTS COME FROM THE MOST IMPORTANT 20% OF YOUR EFFORT.

The fundamentals are the most important things specific to your goals. It's not about doing 100 different exercises, but the vital few that provide the big bang results.

What's ahead in Section IV are exercises that I consider to be the fundamentals for the majority of goals we all have.

After reviewing the key exercises, I'll show you how to maximize a training program depending on the goals you want.

THE PARETO PRINCIPLE

Let's review the **"secret sauce"** to gaining strength – the 80/20 rule, or the Pareto Principle.

My training approach always follows the 80/20 rule, where I focus on the most important 20% of the exercises, chosen to specifically match my primary training objectives.

In other words, at any given time, focus most on what matters – the most important 20%.

If we break things down and put things into "big buckets," then here are the 5 BIG buckets of exercise training that I focus on:

- **Movement (Mobility, Stability, Motor Control)**
- **Bodyweight Training**
- **Kettlebell Training**

- **Powerlifting**
- **Olympic Weightlifting**

We'll cover all this in much more detail in Section IV of the book.

Fitness books can contain literally hundreds of exercises. What you need as a foundation are the most important 20% of the exercises that provide 80% of results.

Instead, *The Edge of Strength* system is focused on helping you discover the 20% of exercises that match your goals. Now, the 20% will change as goals are met and new goals are set.

We'll go over a limited number of exercises – the KEY exercises and lifts that provide the highest value.

That's the difference.

And, then I'm going to suggest additional resources based on the specific areas that are most appropriate for you and where you want to take your training to the next level.

I'll show you why less is more in regard to your training.

Forget the fluff and BS.

We're going to focus on the fundamentals in movement and strength. Don't get distracted, just focus on what matters most for the goals you want – that's your 20%.

Keep this in mind as we discuss the specifics of how to develop strength.

One last time – **FOCUS**.

"More exercise isn't better. Better exercise is better."
-Gray Cook

SECTION IV – DEVELOPING STRENGTH

"Focus on the critical few,
and not the insignificant many."
–Anonymous

CHAPTER 19: STRENGTH STACKING

Absorb what is useful. Discard what is useless.
Add what is uniquely your own."
–Bruce Lee

Now, we get to the important training methods.

Strength Stacking is simply the layering of strength skills on top of one another. It's a continuum primarily based on **skill progression.**

The progression is based on technical proficiency, but your progression doesn't have to go in that order.

This is the exact system I used to advance my training to a new level in recent years. This is my specific progression for strength and performance.

Why do I call this strength stacking?

Once you develop proficiency in one area, then you "stack" on the next progression to advance – if the next stack is appropriate to you and your goals.

Certainly some of the areas can come before others, but I'll outline the most logical progression and explain why this makes sense.

Each progression in the stacking approach is different, but they are all closely related and share common movement principles. They are all connected and fit together.

Strength Stacking is where I spend 90% (or more) of my training efforts. The remaining 10% or less is spent on other proven strength, conditioning, and performance methods.

Do I think most people can move through these progressions and stack them on top of one another?

Definitely. However, it depends on a lot of things.

All progressions may not apply to everyone.

While it would be great for everyone who reads this book to advance through all the progressions and apply them (I'll explain exactly how I use them later in this chapter), it may not be necessary or appropriate.

The main reason is that all progressions may not necessarily fit your goals.

Never do something without being sure it will help you achieve your goals.

In other words, **never do something just to do something.**

Do something because it matches your goals and because you understand how it will contribute to your training and long-term development.

Strength stacking consists of 5 major progressions, which are the 5 major areas of performance training in this book.

The progressions go from lower to higher levels of technical proficiency and skill with higher loads.

Let me share the basic stacking approach for strength and performance, and then explain the why behind each step.

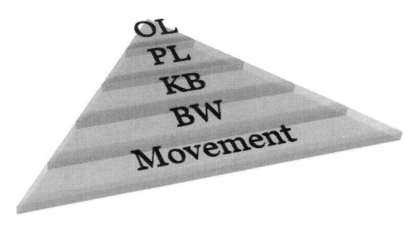

STRENGTH STACKING

- **STACK 1 : MOVEMENT**
- **STACK 2: BODYWEIGHT TRAINING**
- **STACK 3: KETTLEBELL TRAINING**
- **STACK 4: POWERLIFTING**
- **STACK 5: OLYMPIC WEIGHTLIFTING**

Here's a few key similarities and differences to keep in mind about the progressions.

Of course, everything starts with good, quality movement.

SIMILARITIES

- All involve compound, multi-joint movements

- All will significantly contribute to the primary qualities of strength and movement
- All are built around free-form movements
- All have similar principles that can be applied to training

DIFFERENCES

- Progresses to higher loads (exception is Stack 4 and 5)
- Progresses to higher skill levels and technical proficiency
- Progresses from no equipment (or minimal equipment) to more equipment and set-up

LOGICAL ORDER OF PROGRESSION

STACK #1: MOVEMENT

Stack #1 really isn't a strength stack, but a baseline.

Movement is even more foundational than strength. It's where everything starts.

As we've covered, if we don't move well, we can't safely advance to the next progressions in strength and performance.

We must move well before anything else.

Depending on what our "gaps" (or movement deficiencies) are, our training will be structured accordingly.

In other words, **you do what you can with what you have.**

Stack #1 also includes work to address "weak links":

- Movement restrictions
- Weakness
- Immobility
- Instability
- Poor motor control
- Other potential issues

STACK #2: BODYWEIGHT TRAINING (BWT)

After we establish quality, safe movement, next is bodyweight training (BWT).

BWT is the most accessible form of exercise for most people as it requires no equipment (or minimal equipment).

Let's be clear on this progression. It's the fundamental bodyweight movements and exercises, not advanced BWT. Advanced BWT includes various bar exercises (muscle-ups, one-arm pull-ups), gymnastics, or unique feats of strength.

BWT can demand a high level of strength, but **this strength stack refers to the basic and most fundamental BW exercises.**

Stack #2 consists of fundamental variations of:

- Planks
- Push-ups
- Squats
- Pull-ups
- Crawling and rolling
- Ab stabilization work
- Basic "stabilization" exercises
- Handstand work, depending on the individual

We'll cover this in Chapter 20 in much more detail.

STACK #3: KETTLEBELL TRAINING (KBT)

Kettlebell training is the next progression in this "stacking" approach.

We take the movement and strength principles we've learned and apply them to the kettlebell.

And, we progress those training techniques and movement principles even further.

A major advantage of kettlebells is that they allow for increased loads (as compared to BWT), offer different movement patterns, and uniquely allow us to train for both strength and conditioning.

Again, once we have established good baseline movement and a basic demonstration of BWT fundamentals, kettlebells are a logical "next step."

We'll cover kettlebell training in Chapters 21 and 22.

STACK #4: POWERLIFTING (PL)

The next strength stack is the barbell. The fundamental lifts are the "power lifts." The power lifts aren't just for powerlifters, though. They are basic lifts to improve important qualities of strength for all people.

What you need to know is that Stacks #4 and #5 are organized based on technical proficiency only.

Here's what I mean.

Although PL is, without a doubt, technically demanding and requires motor learning, motor skill, and proper coaching, etc., it is not as technical as Stack #5 – Olympic lifting or OL.

PL is moving with maximal loads slowly while OL is lifting with maximal loads as fast and explosively as possible.

As a quick review, the "power lifts" are:

- **Back squat**
- **Bench press**
- **Deadlift**

These 3 lifts are the power lifts.

Personally, I like to mention an essential 4th lift – the **standing military press** – in this group of basic and fundamental lifts.

The lifetime value of these 4 lifts is extremely high.

What do I mean by that?

I mean by doing these lifts for as long as you can, they will provide high value to the quality of your life.

This does not mean you always shoot for maximum strength with these lifts, but that using them with a reasonable load will provide benefit to your life over time.

They will make every person stronger, regardless of age, sex, or background. If all humans performed just these 4 fundamental lifts, we would have a stronger, more powerful, and healthier world.

Are these lifts technical?

Yes, they are.

Like everything in *The Edge of Strength* system, they require great coaching.

They require coaching, a level of understanding, and practice, but they are fundamental lifts that produce results and make us better.

Unfortunately, the bench press (and possibly even the military press) have gotten a bad rap, but with the right coaching and technique, they are extremely valuable and useful lifts for all of us.

Again, these lifts are technical but not as technical as the next progression (weightlifting) for one major reason.

Speed of movement.

Stack #5 introduces more speed and explosiveness to the lifts.

STACK #5: OLYMPIC WEIGHTLIFTING

I believe most would agree that Olympic lifting (OL) is the pinnacle of strength and performance training.

Kettlebells are technical, so is bodyweight training, and so is powerlifting.

But, OL is certainly the most technically demanding because of the speed and explosiveness needed to perform them.

All of the strength stacks require great coaching, but with OL it is critical because of the technical aspects of the lifts.

Many athletes spend years learning and refining these lifts.

I don't want anyone to be discouraged by the challenge of Olympic weight-lifting, but you do have to realize this is not something to dabble with.

Do or do not; there is no try.

The Olympic lifts consist of the barbell snatch and the clean and jerk, along with many key assistance exercises and progressions.

It's amazing when you think about the benefits of just 2 lifts, but they go far and deep, and I believe the upside of OL is endless.

Powerlifting (PL) and OL are often debated – is one better or more beneficial than the other? That depends on the goal.

There are different qualities of strength you are addressing and different demands and unique benefits of each.

One thing is for sure: OL requires more flexibility and mobility to complete the lifts. That's on top of being able to move fast and explosive.

For example, the bottom of the snatch requires a high level of mobility and flexibility in the upper and lower extremities.

And, you need to be able to get under the bar FAST.

Again, PL and OL are different, and both have major benefits relating to strength and performance.

That's why they each represent a separate strength stack.

KEY POINTS ABOUT STRENGTH STACKING

STACKS MAY NOT BE SEQUENTIAL

While this is a continuum, progression, or sequence, you could make arguments for "leapfrogging" over a stack.

It all depends on the goals of the individual, so if someone really wants to get into OL, the strength stacking approach doesn't mean you have to learn kettlebells in order to progress to OL.

Not at all.

That's one reason **stacks are individual categories,** to show how progression can be achieved separately within each.

But, the stacks are organized as a simple way to progress.

Maybe you're already proficient with kettlebells and looking for what's next?

For most people, the next step would be Stack #4 (PL).

The key thing to understand is that Strength Stacking makes sense for most people due to these 3 reasons.

- **Progression of movements**
- **Progression of loads**
- **Progression of technical demands**

But, there are always exceptions.

ALL PROGRESSIONS MUST BE IN ALIGNMENT WITH INDIVIDUAL GOALS

I wanted to make this point clear again.

Strength Stacking is NOT suggesting that everyone must move through these progressions.

The reality is that everything depends on your individual goals.

If a progression is not in alignment with your goals and you cannot answer the question why – then don't do it.

However, the other side is that if you want to continue to evolve your training, develop new skill sets and qualities of strength, and potentially even enter a competition, then Stack #5 is a very valid option.

Strength Stack #5 is a valid option for many reasons.

No matter what you do, always be able to answer the question:

"Why am doing this and how does this contribute to my overall goal?"

STRENGTH STACKS ARE A LOGICAL PROGRESSION

Again, strength stacking progresses from fundamental movements to higher skill, higher demand.

If you take it as it is, it can be very systematic and sequential in terms of progression of movement.

For example, if you can't perform an unloaded bodyweight squat properly, does is make sense to perform a loaded barbell squat?

173

I don't think so.

When in doubt, work on movement first.

Strength Stacking is a simple and logical progression and a system, providing you have good baseline movement.

EACH STACK CAN BE CONSIDERED AN "AREA OF SPECIALIZATION"

The truth is that each area could be considered an area of specialization.

Of course, there's a lot of debate about whether to specialize in training or to keep it generalized (GPP vs. SPP), which was discussed in Chapter 4 – How Strong is Strong Enough?

But, how are you going to get good at anything if you don't specialize or focus?

You can't, and that's why I recommend focusing and even immersing yourself in certain areas, at least for specific time blocks.

I'm sure you've heard the phrase "jack of all trades, master of none."

Personally, I prefer to NOT take that approach.

It may be better to venture far and deep into any of these areas.

As I'll mention later, competitive OL is considered a strength specialty sport, but that doesn't mean you should only engage in OL if you have aspirations to compete.

OL offers tremendous benefits to human strength and performance, even if you have no plans to compete in the sport. And, with the emergence of CrossFit, the popularity of OL has exploded.

The bottom line is that there are many outstanding benefits of OL for many of us, and OL is more accessible to us than we think.

While these areas can be areas of specialization, they also utilize many similar biomechanical principles, which make them all complementary to one another.

That leads me to the final important point about strength stacking.

PROGRESSIONS CAN BE (AND SHOULD BE) COMBINED

The 5 strength stacks can be and should combined.

Bodyweight training and kettlebells fit perfectly together.

Kettlebells complement barbell training.

Bodyweight training (and mobility exercises) naturally benefit barbell training.

My point is that Strength Stacking while it is a progression, does not mean that each area is exclusive to the next.

All of these areas can and should be combined.

The only stacks that could detract from one another in a true periodized approach would be the combination of powerlifting and weightlifting (although they too could be combined in a "hybrid" approach).

HOW I USE STRENGTH STACKING

The way that I use strength stacking is relatively simple.

First, I always make sure that I have Stack #1 – fundamental movement – in order.

I am always self-assessing and ensuring that I can maintain quality movement with the methods I mentioned in Chapter 7.

The way I initially used Strength Stacking was as follows.

When I discovered kettlebells, that tool helped me learn about movement, I made sure I went back and revisited basic movement skills (Stack #1).

Then I re-learned fundamental bodyweight training exercises (Stack #2) as I was learning and implementing kettlebells (Stack #3).

Then, after establishing proficiency with kettlebells, I applied those skills to the barbell with basic barbell lifts and powerlifting (Stack #4).

Then, much later, I progressed to the next level of technical strength development, Olympic weightlifting (Stack #5).

The way I use Strength Stacking today is a little different.

I primarily focus my training on one of 3 areas:

- **Kettlebell Training**
- **Powerlifting (PL)**
- **Olympic Lifting (OL)**

But, I always use the other strength stacks to reinforce the primary training area.

For example, if I am currently doing an OL program, I will still be incorporating Stack #1 and Stack #2 into my approach – and maybe Stack #3, depending on how general or how specialized my programming is at the time.

The bottom line is that I am always combining the training methods represented by each stack, and/or moving up or down through them, depending on my current training goal.

Stacks can be progressed sequentially or combined.

But, Stack #1 (fundamental movement) is always where things begin.

A QUICK SUMMARY

- Movement is the foundation for everything.
- Bodyweight training supports all other strength stacks.
- Kettlebells can be used to support PL and OL
- Bodyweight can be used as a stand-alone strength-training method.
- Kettlebells can be used as a stand-alone.
- PL can be used as a stand-alone.
- OL can be used as a stand-alone.
- All stacks can be combined and integrated for a hybrid strength approach.
- Other tools and methods can be incorporated into Strength Stacking.

In the next few chapters, we'll dive deeper into each strength stack.

We've already covered Stack #1 in Chapter 7, so please refer back to that chapter for Stack #1.

CHAPTER 20: BODYWEIGHT TRAINING

"Fundamental movements are ... fundamental."
–Dan John

STRENGTH STACK # 2

Bodyweight training (BWT) is where it begins after you have established good baseline movement patterns (Stack #1).

Again, we've covered movement in Chapter 7 (Move Well), so we'll start strength training with Stack #2.

As you should understand now, we need to move well THEN move strong.

You can absolutely get strong by using nothing but your own bodyweight. There is nothing more basic and fundamental in strength training than bodyweight training (BWT).

This is the simplest form of strength training and can literally be done anytime or anywhere.

Even though basic bodyweight exercises are fundamental, they can also be considered high performance, such as with gymnastics movements and higher level skills.

But, if you "own" fundamental movements, that qualifies as high performance in my opinion.

BWT can be very simple and is certainly very accessible to all of us.

However, it can also be extremely advanced and high level.

There are some very advanced bodyweight exercises that require a high level of relative strength.

I always include some variation of BWT in my training program, and I typically use it to support the other things I do. It's typically not the focus, although it certainly can be.

For a focused BWT type of programming approach or system, check out books like:

- *Your Body is Your Gym* by Mark Lauren
- *Convict Conditioning* by Paul Wade

- *Never Gymless* by Ross Enamait

The exercises I'll discuss in *The Edge of Strength* serve as a solid foundation for movement and strength.

These are the basics, not necessarily the high level and advanced.

There are several advantages to bodyweight training.

One of the biggest is that it can be incorporated into almost any and every training program.

BWT can also be used for a variety of goals. For example, almost no matter what program I do, I almost always include **pull-ups** because the strict pull-up (or tactical pull-up) offers so much value to a program – **it builds strong lats,** which are important in all the lifts.

While there are many variations of pull-ups, remember that *The Edge of Strength* approach is built around the basic movements. We won't cover every pull-up variation, but, possibly the most important one.

This is not to say the exercise shouldn't be advanced or progressed.

If you remember the SAID principle from Chapter 8, then at some point, we will adapt to the imposed demand.

This is why we need to progress. It's progress or plateau.

BWT is skyrocketing in popularity in the fitness community.

At the time of this writing, BWT is currently one of the top trends in the fitness industry and continues to grow each year.

There's a wide variety of training applications with BWT.

There are new advances and ideas in movement and mobility systems, which is very cool and exciting.

BWT is getting very creative and innovative, but there is also a return to fundamental movements with primitive movements such as crawling, rolling, and rocking.

To learn more about these simple and highly effective movements, I highly recommend the great book, *Original Strength* by Tim Anderson and Geoff Neupert.

This is a book I recommend to everyone because the "OS Reset" is complimentary and beneficial for all.

Both Tim and Geoff have been guests on **The Rdella Training® Podcast** so you can check out those interviews to learn more.

SIMPLICITY

The simplicity of BWT can't be matched.

It requires no equipment, yet produces outstanding results in terms of strength and quality of movement. And, the muscular development can't be ignored either as it's a great way to develop quality, lean muscle.

Can you put on muscle mass with BWT?

Yes, but honestly there are better and more effective methods, barbells and dumbbells, for example.

Many high-level athletes and well-known strength authorities have long used BWT with great success.

There are limitations like anything else, but BWT is a foundational strength and conditioning method. It always has been.

One of the major reasons I like BWT, besides the pure simplicity, is the fact that the principles of movement and technique apply – just as they do with the kettlebell and barbell training.

For example, learning how to use **muscular tension** and **stability** in the push-up or the plank will help with the "set up" of the deadlift or at the top of the kettlebell swing.

The principles of movement carry over to other lifts and exercises.

The positioning and stabilization you learn from BWT will greatly help with the progressions in "strength stacking."

FOCUS

There are an endless number of BWT exercises. *The Edge of Strength* covers only some of the most basic and valuable BWT exercises that I currently use to support my training.

I am not including an endless list of exercises just so you know.

If you are familiar with Pavel Tsatsouline's great book, *Naked Warrior,* you know that the book only covers 2 exercises: the **pistol squat** (single-leg squat) and the **one-arm push-up.**

I highly recommend that book as an extensive book on BWT and the principles of strength development. It goes very deep, beyond just a book on 2 exercises.

We'll just be covering some of the fundamentals, again going back to the 80/20 rule and focusing on what matters most.

Please remember that the goal dictates the tool in the program. Being clear about the training objectives helps you discern which exercises are the right exercises for you.

When your goals are clear, everything else falls into place easily.

Understanding what I just stated is really the key to training success.

Let's quickly review the benefits of BWT:

- No (or minimal) equipment required
- Full-body exercises
- Excellent for different qualities of strength
- Conditioning benefits
- Body composition improvement
- Technical skill improvement
- Sets strong foundation for big lifts
- No barriers to training
- Limits excuses

THE 10 FUNDAMENTALS

Here are 10 of my current fundamental BWT exercises or categories:

1. Bodyweight squat
2. Plank
3. Push-up
4. Pull-up
5. Burpee
6. Ab wheel
7. Handstand work
8. Rolling and Crawling
9. Ring Work
10. Floor work

You and I know there's a lot more to BWT than this, but these fundamentals are a great start to building foundational strength.

BODYWEIGHT SQUAT

BWT really starts with the simple squat.

Before you load a squat, you have to demonstrate a good squat pattern, which begins with a simple bodyweight squat.

It's a great movement prep, conditioning exercise, and movement assessment.

The squat is a fundamental movement, and it's contained in the functional movement screen that we covered in Chapter 7 (although the overhead squat is the variation in the FMS).

Usually, I don't do BW squats in a formal program – primarily because my preference is to load the squat with a barbell or perform squats with kettlebells.

But, I do use the bodyweight squat as a staple in my mobility or movement preparation, so I'm always using a bodyweight squat somewhere in my training.

And, they are very useful for conditioning programs when doing speed squats and also to work on the mechanics of the squat exercise.

Good mechanics start with a simple bodyweight squat. Get your squat pattern right in the bodyweight squat before anything else. It's always beneficial to revisit the proper mechanics of a good squat pattern with an unloaded squat.

Work to keep the spine in good position (back arched), and pull yourself down into the squat with the hips, keeping the knees tracking the toes (no inward collapse of the knees).

Notice the position of your body and how well you move through the movement.

For movement prep, I'll do sets of 5 to 10.

For conditioning, the volume will be much higher.

The advanced version of the bodyweight squat is the **pistol squat,** or one-leg squat. It's exceptional for strength, balance, and full, dynamic range of motion.

One leg is extended out while you squat all the way down on the weight-bearing side. This is considered a very high-level exercise and even a feat of strength.

PLANK

The plank is essential for trunk strength and stability.

It's a great exercise to assess and progress, especially if you've noted weakness in trunk stability.

A quick assessment is the 2-minute plank test.

If you can't hold the plank position for at least 2 minutes, you need spend time and focus on trunk strength and potentially shoulder girdle stabilization.

The floor work exercises will help this.

Most people don't plank with full-body tension, so make sure you remember to squeeze everything when you perform a plank.

Squeeze the glutes, thighs, abs, and get tight while focusing on slow, controlled diaphragmatic breathing.

I typically perform a plank on my elbows, but you can also do the push-up plank position with the elbows fully extended.

They are easy to incorporate into workouts between exercises, say kettlebell swings or goblet squats, for example.

PUSH-UP

The push-up is next because after you've established good trunk strength, the push-up becomes a "moving plank."

The push-up is simple when you learn to use full-body tension and stabilize the shoulders.

To stabilize the shoulders, think of screwing your hands into the floor (or trying to rotate the hands outward – external rotation).

The push-up is a wonderful stability exercise, upper-body developer, and also great for overall strength and conditioning.

How many push-ups?

It all depends on how you're using them in your training program.

In *The Encyclopedia of Underground Strength and Conditioning* by Zach Even-Esh, he wrote about doing **500 push-ups a day.**

He did 50 sets of 10 reps, performing 10 reps every minute for a total time of 50 minutes.

I'm not saying you should do this, but just to give you a reference point.

PULL-UP

The pull-up is an essential upper-body strength exercise.

I do strict pull-ups (or tactical pull-ups), which keep the shoulders safe and effectively use the entire body as the abs are engaged and the spine is in a good position.

A few key points about the tactical pull-up:

- Hands are pronated (palms down or away) on the bar

- Grip the bar approximately shoulder-width or slightly wider
- Pull your shoulders into the sockets to stabilize the shoulder joints
- Tighten your abs by going into the "hollow position"
- Pull yourself up so that your head is above the bar to approximately throat level
- Perform each rep slow and strict

I typically do multiple sets of 5 to 10 in a training program.

The tactical pull-up is an exercise that greatly contributes to other big lifts and improves activation of one of the most important muscles in our body – the lats.

BURPEE

The burpee may be the king of conditioning exercises.

It gets a bad wrap for being so brutal.

Although the burpee is not typically perceived as being technical at all, it actually is very technical.

You get down, push up, and then spring up into a jump.

But, it should be **done with precision** and **controlled movement,** not recklessly rushing through the exercise.

The same stability principles apply in the burpee as the push-up, setting the shoulders and keeping tight throughout the movement.

Transition efficiently through position changes as opposed to flailing your body through the exercise.

If you can do a **100 burpees** total in a training session, you are very well conditioned.

30 burpees is pretty grueling for most people.

A few key tips for the burpee:

- Move through the burpee fast, not sloppy
- Be sure to maintain stability in the trunk and shoulders
- Be efficient
- Own your transitions

AB WHEEL

The ab wheel is one of my favorites because it's so valuable for shoulder and trunk strength. Another great thing is that the ab wheel is inexpensive and portable.

You get on your knees to roll the ab wheel out into an extended position. The advanced version is keeping on your feet and fully rolling out so that your arms and legs are straight.

It's pretty simple, and it's hard to do it wrong.

But, if you have weak trunk strength, it will show up when you try the ab wheel.

And, if you're not used to it, your abs may be sore for days after. The ab wheel forces the abs and entire trunk to contract hard; it's amazing how effective this tool is.

I typically do sets of 10 to 20 reps but start slow if you're not used to it.

HANDSTAND WORK

Handstand work is excellent for shoulder strength, trunk strength, stability, and for training the vestibular system (which helps improve trunk strength).

The **vestibular system** is the inner ear apparatus that is an important sensory system for motion, balance, and spatial orientation.

The first step and most common approach for most is to perform a handstand leaning against a wall.

There are many progressions and variations, but the easiest approach is to find a wall and kick your legs up to hold in a static position. You'll be facing away from the wall when you become inverted.

When you get up against the wall, hold yourself there statically for 10 to 30 seconds – or whatever you feel comfortable with.

If you've never done them, you have to start slow to get accustomed to being inverted, so start slow and don't hang out in a handstand too long.

Make sure to keep your entire body tight and shoulders stable – this is key.

As you become stronger and more accustomed to the position, you will be able to hold longer and even progress into handstand push-ups.

The big thing with this exercise is to understand why you would do it and where it fits.

I like it because of the shoulder and trunk strength benefits, and well as the vestibular system conditioning. It's a very valuable exercise and can be another way to assess shoulder and trunk strength.

And, it just seems to make you feel more dynamic, resilient, and youthful. I don't know why, but that's how I feel with these.

ROLLING AND CRAWLING

I became interested in the benefits of rolling and crawling a few years ago. For me, it started when I attended a workshop with Geoff Neupert and then began reading the work of Tim Anderson.

CRAWLING

Benefits of crawling:

- Strengthens the shoulders
- Strengthens the trunk
- Conditioning
- Reflexive strength (ties in trunk stabilizers)
- Improves movement and mobility
- Excellent movement preparation prior to training

For more on the benefits of crawling and rolling (which I'll discuss next), I would highly recommend the book *Original Strength* by Tim Anderson and Geoff Neupert.

Crawling can be used as movement preparation, part of a program, as a conditioning component, or a variety of other ways. I prefer **Spiderman crawls** as my preferred crawl.

Both crawling and rolling are extremely valuable for total-body strength and movement.

Crawling represents the foundational strength we should all have. And since it's easy to do, there's no reason not to include it somewhere in your training.

ROLLING

Get on the ground, and roll around. Yes, it can be that easy, but there are different ways to roll that can be quite challenging.

I like to use **segmental rolls** for movement preparation, mobility, and trunk strength.

Segmental rolls are when I use my upper body to initiate the rolls, then I'll use the lower body to initiate the rolls (upper-body segment, then lower-body segment).

Rolling has similar benefits to crawling and tends to do wonders for our bodies. It strengthens the body, improves movement and mobility, and gets us on the ground for our ground work (or floor work).

Why roll? To move better and get stronger overall.

If you have mobility issues, try rolling and crawling for a couple of weeks using the methods by Tim Anderson.

Do his simple "reset" and see if it doesn't almost magically clear up some things. You have nothing to lose, but you sure can gain a lot from a "reset."

RING WORK

Ring work is using set of gymnastics rings, which I use on my pull-up bar.

I love gymnastics rings for shoulder girdle strength and stability. Typically, what I'll do is either static holds or ring dips.

Ring dips are obviously more challenging and difficult, but they are exceptional for the chest, shoulders, and arms.

One of the key benefits of the holds or dips is the muscle activation of the rotator cuff. The rotator cuff consists of 4 muscles in your shoulder joint that hold the ball (the humeral head) in the socket (the glenoid).

The static holds and dynamic movement with rings get the rotator cuff, lats, scapular stabilizers, and everything else in the shoulder girdle to fire at a high level.

A few sets of static holds or a few sets of 5 to 8 ring dips, and you may be amazed at how strong your upper body becomes. And they're exceptional for shoulder health.

Start with holds, progress to dips.

FLOOR WORK

This is the only thing on the list that is not an exercise, but a **category of exercises** that greatly contribute to trunk strength and stability.

I like these exercises as part of a movement preparation program or as a prehab/rehab approach.

The key exercises are listed here for your reference, but check out Rdella-Training.com to learn more about them.

- Deadbugs (the exercise)
- Bird Dogs
- Supine Hip Bridges
- Supine Breathing and Stabilization
- Unweighted Turkish get ups
- Transitional movement patterns

KEY POINTS ABOUT BWT

First, this is just a quick overview of BWT, an intro to what I consider to be some of the fundamentals.

These 10 things are currently the foundation of my bodyweight training programming, and they fit into the other things I do without detracting from anything.

This is not to say this all I do or all you should do.

These are what I consider to be the foundation of strong bodyweight training. Obviously, there's a lot more to BWT than what I mention in this chapter.

For more progressions and programming, definitely check out the great books I've recommended and consider what could be your fundamentals.

No matter what, stick to the basics.

"Movement isn't important until you can't."
-Gray Cook

CHAPTER 21: KETTLEBELLS – THE HANDHELD GYM

"Kettlebells are a different version of strong."
–Charlie Weingroff

STRENGTH STACK #3

A complete training system with a simple, proven, and highly effective tool that provides a high level of strength and conditioning – that's the kettlebell.

The kettlebell is just a tool. But, it's a damn good tool.

This was the tool that changed my entire training philosophy.

It was the kettlebell that got me back into barbell training.

It was also the tool that helped me re-discover movement and performance.

If you think it's similar to a dumbbell, then you haven't attended a workshop, seminar, or certification yet to learn how and why the kettlebell is different.

Not a problem as I'll try to explain how it's unique and different here, but to understand what I mean, you have to pick one up and experience it for yourself. You have to learn how to use it the right way.

The first thing I want to point out is there are different styles of kettlebell training.

For example, there is **Girevoy Sport,** the competitive style of kettlebells which is entirely different from the kettlebell training I'll tell you about, which is the **hardstyle technique** of kettlebell training.

We have many tools and choices to optimize our health and performance today. Some tools are better than others. The kettlebell is definitely one of the better ones.

The kettlebell is an amazing tool. But, it's only amazing when you learn how to use it properly.

The beauty of kettlebells is in the fundamental exercises, which I'll cover in next chapter. We can progress beyond these basics with a lot of options, but it always comes back to the fundamentals.

Build a strong foundation with the fundamentals.

MY FIRST EXPERIENCE WITH KETTLEBELLS

I happen to see a workshop advertised in South Florida to learn about kettlebell training. The claim was that by attending this one-day workshop, the attendee would have a solid grasp of Russian-style kettlebell training (hardstyle technique).

Andrea DuCane and that workshop changed my life.

I was skeptical about what I would learn by attending because I thought I had a good sense of how to use the tool already (even though I had no formal training with it).

But I attended since I figured I would at least pick up a few things that could help me progress my training.

It wasn't long into the workshop that I discovered there was so much more to kettlebell training than I ever imagined.

Actually, I was blown away by how much power and effectiveness there was with this tool.

I realized I didn't know what I was doing and the experience was humbling, to say the least. But, that workshop and that style of training completely aligned with my personal philosophy about training.

Move well, get strong, and always keep improving.

The hardstyle approach (Russian style) is about moving well with proper biomechanics and optimizing joint position.

Hardstyle is about moving with power, efficiency, and explosiveness.

There are different styles of kettlebell training, but the hardstyle approach made the most sense to me with my background as a PT. After that workshop, I continued to discover that kettlebell training was truly a revolutionary way to train and achieve a variety of benefits.

If you already train with kettlebells, you know exactly what I mean.

And, if you're new to kettlebells, then I'll help you discover the art and science of kettlebells to get great results.

That workshop taught me that what I had been doing for the last several months was all wrong. I was humbled. Even though I'd been training for so many years, I hadn't yet been properly trained with kettlebells.

I realized I didn't know as much about movement and performance as I thought I did. And, sadly, my kettlebell technique was not too good.

Kettlebells are about movement, first and foremost.

When the tool is used properly, you'll move better, move stronger, and the tool delivers proven and powerful results.

I'm not saying kettlebells are all you should do, and this is why I've found such great success with the Strength Stacking approach.

What I am saying is that kettlebells could be a core component to your training for the rest of your life. The tool can certainly be complimentary to other things you do.

Strength Stack #3 can be the main focus of your training or it can be supportive. How kettlebells fit into your strength training program depends on goals, as we've covered.

We're all looking for simple solutions to get powerful results.

Kettlebells offer the proven combination of **simplicity and results.**

WHAT MAKES KETTLEBELLS DIFFERENT?

Imagine a tool that you could use to address the vast majority of your health and fitness goals.

A tool to forge an athletic, resilient, dynamic body.

Imagine that this tool was proven, powerful and could be easily stored and transported anywhere you wanted.

How would you feel if this wasn't some silly gimmick or fitness fad, but a simple tool that's been used by athletes and legendary strong men for many centuries?

This is the kettlebell.

The kettlebell is just a cannon ball with a handle that is manipulated in very specific ways to address high levels of fitness and performance.

Yet, how you use this tool will be incredibly valuable, humbling, and rewarding. You can always get better and deepen your skills, even with the basics.

In a cluttered fitness industry full of fads, gimmicks and nonsense – kettlebell training is the real deal.

Something about the shape, design, and how you use the tool makes it different. And unlike anything else.

One of the main problems in fitness today is too many choices. Too many gadgets, exercise methods, too many programs, too much misinformation, and quite frankly, too much flat-out nonsense.

We all want variety and want to do different things to gain strength; I understand that. But, we have to remember that 80% of our results comes from the most important 20% of what we do.

I've been fortunate to speak with and learn from many of the top strength and conditioning coaches in world, people who I highly respect and have been honored to speak with one-on-one.

This includes great strength coaches and experts like:

- Pavel Tsatsouline
- Kelly Starrett
- Dan John
- Geoff Neupert
- Gray Cook
- Brett Jones
- Dr. Stuart McGill

They all agree that the kettlebell is an effective and powerful training tool unlike any other.

A QUICK KETTLEBELL REVIEW

The tool is brutally simple.

Again, it's just a cannon ball with an offset handle, but that's what makes it different.

The recent popularity and growth has made it seem like it's a new tool on the scene, but it's not.

For me, the kettlebell was the catalyst for where I am today and helping me rediscover human potential and a whole new level of strength and conditioning.

THE KETTLEBELL IS A SIMPLE, UNIQUE TOOL THAT CAN HELP MANY PEOPLE ACHIEVE A VARIETY OF FITNESS GOALS.

Applying the movement principles I've learned from kettlebell training has taught me so much more about how to improve my barbell training techniques.

Here are the key benefits of kettlebell training:

- Improves strength
- Enhances flexibility
- Improves mobility
- Helps movement and motor control
- Skill development
- Builds a high level of cardiovascular conditioning
- Accelerates fat loss
- Builds quality, lean muscle

- Mental toughness
- Develops full body power and explosiveness
- Forges a more athletic looking body
- Boosts confidence and mental state
- Supports other training methods (barbells, bodyweight training)

Depending on training goals, it will be a larger part of my programming or a lesser part, but it will always be a part of the program.

If you haven't discovered the tool, you owe it to yourself to learn how.

And, if you have discovered it, this book will confirm what you already know and will help you nail the fundamentals.

Learn how to perform a **kettlebell swing** properly, and always work on improving. Learn how to do a **Turkish get-up** properly, and always work on improving.

Immerse yourself in these exercises and **learn from someone that is certified** and knows what they are doing with a kettlebell – this is a requirement, not a suggestion.

Once you have a solid foundation with the fundamental exercises, which we'll review in the next chapter, you could begin by doing simple training sessions like this.

TRAINING SESSION EXAMPLE

- 15 minutes of kettlebell swings (*rest as needed during the 15 minutes, and log your total reps)
- 5 minutes of continuous get-ups under moderate load (switching hands every rep, going slow and steady, and "owning" the movements and transitions)

This is such a simple training template that offers incredible benefits, and it's great for beginner or advanced athletes.

If you're ever in doubt about what to do, do this.

Again, simple, but not easy. Effective strength training never is.

THE RIGHT WAY TO USE KETTLEBELLS

The truth is that kettlebells require high-quality instruction if you really want to maximize the benefits of the tool. This is no different from learning how to properly use a barbell, which we'll discuss soon.

If you're brand new to kettlebells, it's highly recommended to get at least a session from a qualified instructor, or use the resources I'll mention at the end of the book.

The first step would be to find a qualified kettlebell instructor.

This is a requirement to get the best training in the safest, most efficient way possible.

At this time, I'm a StrongFirst level II kettlebell instructor (SFGII) and have been for the last few years. My recommendation would be to go to Strong-First.com and look for an instructor in your area.

StrongFirst is where you'll find the current techniques and methods taught by Pavel Tsatsouline.

Another option for you to learn hardstyle kettlebell training is through DragonDoor.com.

I can't speak too much about the other organizations or certifications, simply because I have not gone through their programs, but I am familiar with them.

As I've mentioned, hardstyle kettlebell training most aligned with my own training philosophy and movement principles, based on my background as a physical therapist and someone obsessed with human movement.

Pavel's techniques aligned best with my philosophy.

The first step to finding the kettlebell training method that works for you is to find out if you have a certified instructor close to you.

If you don't have anyone close, don't rule out **online coaching** as a viable option.

Live coaching is best, but online coaching definitely works. It's better than no coaching, and you can get valuable feedback about your technique and how you move.

Another option are some of the outstanding books and DVD products that are listed in the resource section of this book.

I'd recommend these regardless, as they are all outstanding products that will help with your learning of the proper use of kettlebells.

Additionally, I wrote an extremely comprehensive article on kettlebell training. In that article, you will find many more resources and answers to your questions, so I recommend checking that out.

The article is titled **"The Ultimate Guide to Kettlebell Training"** on Rdel-laTraining.com.

Or you can go here:

http://rdellatraining.com/the-ultimate-guide-to-kettlebell-training

In the next chapter, we'll get specific with fundamental exercises, the kettlebell essentials. Of course, you'll need kettlebells to put those into practice.

Kettlebell size guidelines depend on current strength, training experience, bodyweight, gender, age, and other factors.

If we keep the kettlebell recommendations as "general," then here are the kettlebell sizes:

- *Women: 8kg (18 lb.) kettlebell (or up to 12 kg – 26 pounds)*
- *Men: 16kg (35 lb.) kettlebell (or up to 24 kg – 53 pounds)*

And, I've been recommending the Rogue kettlebells for years now, but there are many high-quality kettlebells on the market.

CHAPTER 22: KETTLEBELL ESSENTIALS

"The kettlebell swing is the center of the conditioning universe."
–David Whitley

I covered why kettlebell training is a great training option for many of us.

Now, we'll cover the kettlebell fundamental exercises and why these can be the foundation for great training.

We'll go into more detail about how to do these exercises and spend more time understanding the importance of great technique.

Even if you're advanced with kettlebells, I'd highly encourage you to read through this material and look for key insights to improve your kettlebell skills.

Everyone can always improve and get better, no matter where you are in strength progressions.

KETTLEBELL FUNDAMENTALS

The kettlebell fundamentals in hardstyle kettlebell training comes down to the following:

- **Deadlift (to establish the hip hinge)**
- **Kettlebell swing**
- **Goblet squat**
- **Turkish get up**
- **Strict press**
- **Clean**
- **Snatch**

The feet must be stable and planted into the ground when training with kettlebells.

With that understanding, you should train in bare feet or with a flat, stable sole shoe. Converse Chuck Taylor's or similar minimalist shoes are the best.

What you don't want are cushioned running shoes that are unstable and soft. This is unsafe as it will not provide a solid base to perform the kettlebell ballistics (fast movements) or the grinds (slow movements).

BIOMECHANICAL MATCHED BREATHING

Before getting to the kettlebell movements, we have to cover the importance of breathing.

This is key to the kettlebell swing and all the kettlebell exercises for power, efficiency, and safety.

If you want to crush it with kettlebells, master your breathing.

Here's how it works.

What you will be doing is appropriately called biomechanical matched breathing (or power breathing). What this means is the breath matches the force production during the exercise.

For example, as the kettlebell swings forward, you will need to exert significant force to propel the kettlebell.

This means you will be exhaling and matching the breath to the movement as you swing the bell forward. This tightens the abs and stabilizes the spine. This also **gives you unbelievable power.**

Conversely, as the kettlebell comes back between your legs, you will now inhale.

Ideally, you will want to learn how to inhale through your nose and exhale through your mouth in a controlled breathing technique.

Essentially, use a "hissing" technique as you exhale and propel the kettlebell forward.

Why hiss?

To allow air to be expelled slowly until the swing is complete at the top, where you expel the remaining air at maximum force production.

This specific breathing technique makes the swing extremely powerful and efficient.

Think of throwing a punch.

If, by chance, you have a background in martial arts, this will be easy because you already know how to use this breathing technique to maximize force production.

At the end of the punch, maximal exhalation occurs giving you the extra power precisely when you need it.

This will take some practice, but if you use this technique, you'll understand how powerful and effective it is.

THE HIP HINGE PATTERN

Hardstyle kettlebell training has to begin with the hip hinge pattern. Before attempting a kettlebell swing or even a deadlift, it's very important to hinge properly from the hips.

The hinge is exactly what it sounds like – a movement that occurs at the hips while keeping a neutral or straight spine.

The hips hinge and the body moves. It's simple but often misunderstood.

Here's the 3 steps to perform a proper hip hinge.

STEP 1

In a standing position, place your hands in the fold of your hips.

Keep the back tall and in a neutral position.

STEP 2

Drive the hips back while allowing the shoulders to come forward, hinging or pivoting from the hips.

The hands should sink into the crease of the hips.

STEP 3

Bend the knees slightly but not excessively. This is the difference between a hinge and a squat. It's important to note that the kettlebell swing is NOT a squat pattern, but a hinge pattern.

A dowel rod or inexpensive PVC pipe is a great way to provide feedback on the proper hip hinge movement.

Place the rod behind your back so that it is in contact from your head to your pelvis. Now, hinge by driving the hips back, and allow the shoulders to come forward and keep the contact of the rod with your spine.

This is an excellent technique to practice the hip hinge.

BIG MISTAKE

By far, one of the biggest mistakes with the kettlebell swing is not hinging properly.

Many online videos demonstrate incorrect form and show a squat movement pattern as opposed to a hinge movement pattern. Be careful with what you see on YouTube!

Once you establish a proper hinge, then it's safe to begin to load the pattern with a deadlift.

A kettlebell is an ideal way to begin a loaded hip hinge pattern. That's why the kettlebell deadlift is the critical first exercise in the kettlebell fundamentals. After properly learning the deadlift, then comes the kettlebell swing.

The kettlebell swing is a very deceiving exercise because it can be perceived as a very simple exercise.

However, simple does not mean easy.

There are a lot of technical nuances to pay attention to.

Performing the kettlebell swing correctly will require proper motor learning and proper breathing with a thorough understanding of how to perform the swing correctly.

Proper breathing maximizes the benefits and is a crucial part of kettlebell training.

Learn to hiss, and take your performance to the next level. Ok, let's get back to the deadlift.

As I cover the essential kettlebell exercises, please refer to RdellaTraining. com for additional training resources, including video training on the YouTube channel.

You can go to **YouTube.com/RdellaTraining**.

DEADLIFT

The fundamental kettlebell exercises begin with a good deadlift.

It's not about the weight; it's about the movement.

This is worth repeating.

The kettlebell deadlift is about movement, not maximum strength.

We all need to establish a good hip hinge pattern, and that's why the kettlebell deadlift is an important and valuable exercise, especially when getting started with this training tool.

It's also good to go back to the exercise to engrain the pattern, even as an experienced kettlebell lifter.

This is in contrast is the barbell deadlift (DL), which we'll cover in the next chapter. The barbell DL is about maximum strength and power as we load the barbell with much heavier weight.

The kettlebell deadlift is about getting a proper movement pattern established before we progress to **the athletic fat-burning machine otherwise known as the kettlebell swing.**

Key considerations for the kettlebell deadlift:
- Hinge at the hips and keep a neutral spine
- Keep the lats tight

- Move through the movement slowly
- Begin to practice biomechanical breathing
- Keep a slight bend at the knee
- Squeeze the glutes at the top

Here's how to do the kettlebell deadlift.

STEP 1

Position the kettlebell between your feet. Keep the bell approximately parallel to the heels so that the kettlebell is positioned slightly back in your stance.

STEP 2

Your feet will be approximately shoulder-width apart with the toes turned slightly out.

STEP 3

From a standing tall position, initiate the movement by driving your hips back while keeping the back flat.

The knees will bend slightly as you move and reach down toward the kettlebell to grab the handle.

STEP 4

You should be hinging properly with a neutral spine until your hands come into contact with the kettlebell.

At this point, you'll grab the bell and drive your heels through the floor.

Stand up quickly into an upright position, driving the hips forward. Exhale as you come to the standing position.

STEP 5

From a standing tall position, begin to hinge again, driving the hips back and lowering the kettlebell back to the ground.

Place the kettlebell back in starting position safely.

It's essential to start, transition, and finish the entire movement in a fluid, dynamic, and safe movement pattern to establish a proper loaded hip hinge.

Hopefully, this point is very clear by now.

GOBLET SQUAT

The goblet squat (GS) is a dynamic exercise for strength, conditioning, mobility, and stability.

It requires a great degree of hip and knee movement as well as mobility.

Let's not confuse the goblet squat with a barbell squat. The barbell squat is a much more effective exercise for total-body strength.

The goblet squat, on the other hand, is beneficial for movement, mobility, and general strength and conditioning purposes. It's not a maximum strength developer, and no one claims that it is.

Here are some key considerations for the goblet squat:

- Keep a neutral spine
- Feet are firmly planted
- Knees in alignment with toes – prevent valgus collapse (knees in)
- Pause briefly at the bottom of the squat
- Drive up with proper breathing – exhalation
- Hips and shoulder rise simultaneously as a unit
- Keep tight and stable throughout the movement

Keep in mind that this is usually very difficult to do incorrectly. The limitation would be the inability to squat properly or demonstrate sufficient mobility.

Here's how to do the goblet squat.

STEP 1

Grab the kettlebell by the handle or horns, and hold it directly in front of your chest.

STEP 2

Get your stance right.

You will assume a shoulder-width stance and point your toes out just slightly.

This is your standard squatting stance.

STEP 3

Initiate the movement by sitting down or pulling back with your hips and inhale on the descent.

You want to think about initiating the movement with your hip flexors as you pull down into the squat position.

STEP 4

Descend slowly and with control and stability while keeping your back flat or arched.

Think of maintaining "tall spine" position.

You want to have your feet rooted firmly on the ground with your weight sitting back on your heels, not on your toes.

As you descend down into the bottom of the squat (or the hole), you want to maintain the tall spine or keep a slight extension in your low back.

At no point in the bottom do you want to come into a forward flexed or hunched position.

STEP 5

Pause momentarily in the bottom of the squat.

Your elbows should be the inside of your thighs.

STEP 6

You want to exhale as you ascend up with a strong, powerful movement.

When you stand up, be sure that your hips and shoulders ascend at the same time.

Get tall, exhale, and squeeze the glutes at the top or finish position.

KETTLEBELL SWING (RUSSIAN STYLE)

Now you're ready for the kettlebell swing, the fat-burning athlete builder.

This is the foundation of all kettlebell exercises.

It's critical to get the swing right before progressing to the other ballistic exercises, such as the kettlebell clean and kettlebell snatch.

If you don't have the swing down, you don't have kettlebell training.

Again, we start with establishing the proper hip hinge and a proper dead-lift before progressing to the kettlebell swing, just to be clear.

TWO-ARM SWING

We're going to start off with the **two-arm kettlebell swing.**

That means you're grasping the kettlebell with two hands and not just one.

After establishing the two-arm kettlebell swing, we'll cover the one-arm kettlebell swing as well, although essentially it follows the same movement pattern.

The difference is that the one-arm swing is challenged differently than the two-arm kettlebell swing.

Here are the key things to keep in mind, and then we'll take the swing step by step:

- Keep the back flat.

- Keep the feet planted firmly on the ground.
- Shoulders are packed (shoulder joints and shoulder blades set and stable).
- Keep the kettlebell handle above the knee on the back swing.
- At the top of the swing, the body forms a straight line from the feet through the head (neutral spine and not hyperextended).
- Kettlebell is elevated to approximately shoulder level.
- Use biomechanical matched breathing – exhale as the bell goes forward.
- Abs and glutes are contracted at the top of the swing.

Let's cover the essential steps in kettlebell swing mechanics.

STEP 1

Assume a shoulder-width stance with the toes pointing slightly out. This is a basic squat stance.

STEP 2

Position the kettlebell in front of you where you can reach out to fully extend the arms comfortably.

Grab the kettlebell handle, and tilt the bell back so that the kettlebell and the arms are in complete alignment.

STEP 3

When you're getting set in the position to hike the kettlebell back, you are essentially doing a hip hinge in your set-up to get in position to hike the kettlebell back.

Think about keeping the spine neutral and in a straight or tall position.

When you are set to begin the swing, you will be set up with your body slightly behind the kettlebell. The hamstrings will be loaded. The back will be flat.

STEP 4

As you begin the kettlebell swing, you will hike the kettlebell back aggressively between your legs.

Hike the kettlebell high with your forearms hitting the inside of your thighs.

Think about this as if you were hiking a football and bringing the football high up into your groin.

STEP 5

Once the kettlebell has been hiked and is in the back position, the next step is to explosively drive the hips forward to propel the kettlebell to approximately shoulder height.

This step is the key to maximizing performance with the kettlebell swing.

It's the **explosive hip drive** and the fast movement of the hips that will allow the kettlebell to float effortlessly to approximately shoulder height.

In the Russian-style swing, you are not taking the kettlebell overhead but are projecting the kettlebell to be horizontal with the ground.

STEP 6

At the top of the swing, the kettlebell is approximately shoulder height.

You want to think about the tall spine position. Do not excessively extend back into lumbar hyperextension.

You want to be very tall and straight at the top of the swing.

STEP 7

The importance of the explosive hip drive and the quickness of the kettlebell swing movement can't be emphasized enough.

You must explosively drive the hips to propel the kettlebell horizontally at the top of the swing.

It's a fast and explosive movement.

ONE-ARM SWING

The next exercise we'll cover will be the one-arm kettlebell swing, essentially the same movement pattern as the two-arm swing we just reviewed.

The only difference is the challenge at the top of the swing. The body will be challenged to rotate to the opposite side that the kettlebell is held.

There will be an increased force at the top of the swing that will pull you or try to rotate you to the opposite side of the kettlebell.

If you're doing a one-arm kettlebell swing holding the kettlebell on the left side, at the top of the swing, the force will try to rotate you toward the right side.

What you want to do is counteract this force by staying strong and stable in the top position.

You will want to resist the right-side rotation, and a good way that I've found to do that is with a good drill called **touch the bell.**

When you're holding the kettlebell on the left side, as you're swinging forward with the kettlebell at the top of the swing, you will reach over with your right hand and just tap the kettlebell at the top of the swing.

What this does is help to square the shoulders at the top of the swing.

Again, you want to **resist the rotation** and maintain a tall upright posture with a one-hand swing.

The key benefit with the one-arm swing is being able to perform a higher volume of repetitions.

The difference is that when you do high-volume reps with a two-arm swing, the limiting factor, assuming you are conditioned appropriately, will ultimately be your grip strength.

If you're swinging a heavy kettlebell for high-volume repetitions, **grip failure** will often limit further volume with the two-arm kettlebell swing.

The one-arm swing allows you to switch hands – for example, doing ten reps on the left, ten reps on the right – and repeat the sequence for multiple sets.

This is giving your grip strength a rest in between those ten reps, which allows for much more volume than two-arm swings.

There are benefits to both the one-arm swing and the two-arm swing, which is why I use them both. They are both essential, unique, and beneficial in any strength and conditioning program.

Essentially they are both built the same way, as far as the mechanics of the explosive hip drive.

One final point is that the one-arm swing also allows you to transition into other single-arm ballistic exercises that we'll cover, which include the kettlebell clean and the kettlebell snatch.

Therefore, good technique with the one-arm swing allows you to better transition or learn the clean and snatch. We'll discuss them soon.

THE TURKISH GET UP (TGU)

Next up is the Turkish get-up (TGU) which is one of the most valuable exercises in physical training. It's been around for many decades and has been used by some of the legends and pioneers in strength and performance.

When I say that this exercise is for every athlete, fitness enthusiast, and human – I mean it.

It's an exercise we should be doing for the rest of our lives.

The TGU is simply getting up from the ground using a kettlebell in a slow, deliberate movement.

Of course, there's a lot more to the technique than that, but that's basically what the TGU is.

It's an extremely powerful and effective exercise demonstrating a high level of mobility and stability, and it offers value to all of us.

The truth is that it's an exercise we should be doing for as long as we possibly can to maximize human movement and functional capacity.

Most experts agree we need to spend more time on the ground, since as we age, we'll want to do everything we can to NOT end up there (in other words, preventing falls).

Another great benefit is that the TGU can be programmed into almost every exercise program and enhances performance due to the significant benefits of the exercise.

The TGU could be used in a powerlifter's program and a weightlifter's program. I'm not saying this would be the focus, but it would be useful as an accessory exercise or for movement and mobility work.

The TGU just seems to help everything else.

The Turkish get-up is an exercise that I believe should be done with a kettlebell, as opposed to other tools.

It can be done with a dumbbell.

It can even be done with a barbell.

But, the kettlebell, due to the shape and design, makes it an ideal tool for performing the Turkish get-up.

Before even starting with a kettlebell and loading the movement pattern of the Turkish get-up, it's very important to perform the movement from the floor to standing up tall and going back down to the floor without weight.

LEARN THE MOVEMENT FIRST, AND THEN LOAD THE MOVEMENT.

To see these detailed steps, please refer to the videos on my YouTube Channel.

YouTube.com/RdellaTraining

Here are a few key things to remember.

- The elbow and wrist is always straight on the side that you hold the kettlebell.
- Keep the shoulders packed and stable throughout the movement.

- Make sure to keep the heels planted during transitions – feet stable.
- Keep the arm holding the kettlebell vertical throughout the movement.
- The entire spine should be in good alignment as you go through the transitions.

Now with that said, let's cover the steps involved in performing a Turkish get-up.

STEP 1

You will be positioned in a side-lying position.

For this example, the Turkish get-up will be done with the **kettlebell in the right hand.**

You're going to lay on your right side, the hips and knees flexed. Essentially, lay down in a fetal-like position on your side with the spine in a neutral or straight position.

STEP 2

Next, you're going to grab the kettlebell and roll over onto your back.

You want to prevent the shoulder from being excessively stretched anteriorly.

What you're going to do is grab the kettlebell with both hands and roll over as a unit so that you're on your back.

STEP 3

Press the kettlebell with both hands, and now you're holding the kettlebell in the right hand so that the arm is straight.

The left arm and leg are slightly away out to the side.

The right hip and knee are flexed, and the left leg is straight.

This is the starting position, lying on the floor.

On the side you're holding the kettlebell, make sure that you pull the shoulder blade back into the ground, pulling the shoulder into the socket so that it's tight and stable. This is known as packing the shoulder.

STEP 4

Once you are in proper position on the floor with the shoulder set, you will then come up onto the elbow.

Drive or push away onto the floor from the left elbow, and drive through your right heel.

You want to think about keeping strong and stable through the spine.

The TGU is essentially driving away from the floor, with the extremities, while keeping a rigid or stable spine.

STEP 5

Now, you're positioned up on your elbow, holding the kettlebell up with your right arm. Keep a tall chest (chest up).

Looking up at the kettlebell, simply push up on your left to come up onto the hand from the elbow.

STEP 6

Next, you have 2 options to bring the leg through: the **low sweep** or the **high bridge.**

For the low sweep technique, simply sweep the left leg back through your body so you will be positioned in a half-kneeling position.

Or you can do what I like to do, which is called a high bridge.

In the high bridge, you will raise the pelvis high in the air so that the trunk and spine become rigid. Use the hip drive and glutes to extend the hips and spine before bringing the left leg through, coming back onto the half-kneeling position.

I should clarify that the left hand is still on the ground, so you are on the left knee and left hand.

STEP 7

Once you're in this half-kneeling position with the kettlebell in your right hand, you have weight that is on your left knee and on your left hand.

Now pivot and square off facing forward into the full half-kneeling position – essentially a lunge position - the left hand now comes off the floor.

Look straight ahead.

STEP 8

The finish of the TGU from the floor is to lunge forward, exhaling as you come forward while holding the kettlebell in a lockout position overhead.

That would be the finish position, the standing position of the Turkish get-up.

To complete the get-up, simply reverse these steps to get back down.

Take a big step back, come down onto the knee, etc. Again, I highly recommend checking out my **YouTube video to see** these step-by-step progressions.

When you get back down on the ground on your back, you're going to lower the kettlebell into the ribcage. Roll to the side that's holding the kettlebell, and place the bell back on the ground.

All of these steps would be one repetition of the TGU.

The TGU can be perceived as a complex movement or exercise.

It actually is not – when each of these steps is broken down individually.

This is how I teach the TGU, breaking it down step by step.

We get the movements for step #1 and step #2 down first so that they become automatic. That means they're safe and fluid.

Then we will advance to the next step.

We keep going through step #1, step #2, step #3 until those movements are learned.

Then we will continue to stack on the additional steps so that the TGU is learned to be performed as one movement.

The TGU is easy to learn when it is broken down into smaller steps. This is the key.

The TGU is not meant to be rushed.

It is a slow and deliberate movement.

The proper way that it should be done is to pause between each transition. Don't rush through it. Perform the movement slower than you think you should, and own each movement and each transition along the way.

The benefits of the TGU are significant in terms of mobility, stability, strength, and movement. In particular, the shoulder health benefits are outstanding.

This is one of the most effective, dynamic shoulder strengthening exercises we have available to us.

Unfortunately, the TGU is an exercise that is not done by the majority of the population due to lack of understanding and possibly the unconventional nature of the exercise.

However, the **TGU is as close to magical** as any exercise I've ever experienced.

My good friend and physical therapist Chuck Mutschler recently said something that was absolutely brilliant.

He said his big goal was 70 at 70 – to be able to perform a 70-pound Turkish get up at age 70.

Can you imagine the strength and resiliency necessary for this goal?

B.H.A.G. GOAL = 70 LB. TGU @ 70

It doesn't have to be that number. Think about what a strong, powerful TGU would be for you now, and then make that your B.H.A.G. For example, it could be a "50 @ 70" or "35 @ 70," whatever feels reasonable and attainable for you.

Regardless of what number you choose, the TGU is one of the most valuable exercises for every athlete and fitness enthusiast.

THE CLEAN

The kettlebell clean is another powerful movement.

It's exceptional as an explosive exercise, a powerful exercise, with the added benefit of improving arm strength and explosive hip drive and power.

Master kettlebell instructor Dave Whitley has called the kettlebell clean a swing that finishes in the rack position. That's basically what it is.

THE RACK POSITION

The rack position is where the kettlebell sits tight on the front of your body.

The kettlebell is resting on the outside of your forearm, but the hand is positioned below your chin in front of the clavicle or in front of the chest for men.

For women, the rack position is going to be positioned slightly out to the side a little bit more, based on the anatomy of the breast tissue.

It is very important to get the rack position situated correctly.

The elbow will be down into your side. This will be a very strong, stable, and secure position with the kettlebell resting on the outside of the forearm and the hand, upper arm, and forearm all in proper position.

This is the rack position, and this is the position that the clean will finish in. It's also the position that the kettlebell press will begin from, so it's very important.

Here are key things to know about the clean:

- The same principles from the swing apply to the clean.
- Keep the wrist straight during the clean.
- The path of the kettlebell matters – keep the bell close to your body.

There is contact of the kettlebell on the forearm at the top of the clean, but this should occur without major impact, in other words – there should be no "banging."

Now, let's go through how to execute the kettlebell clean.

STEP 1

Get set up properly. The start position will be the same as the one-hand kettlebell swing.

Position the kettlebell out in front of you, and aggressively hike the kettlebell back between your legs in a high position in your groin.

STEP 2

You're going to explosively drive with the hips elevating the kettlebell up to the rack position.

Here's the difference with the clean compared to the one-arm swing: the path of the kettlebell will be positioned closer to your body with the clean. In the one arm swing, the kettlebell is projected far away from your body.

The clean comes almost essentially right up your body, and the kettlebell lands safely or is positioned safely on the outside of the forearm.

There should be absolutely no banging as the bell is repositioned at finish of the clean.

Let me repeat that.

There should be absolutely no banging of the kettlebell as the kettlebell lands or positions on the outside of the forearm.

The kettlebell clean is a movement that requires practice and a "feel" or groove. In other words, it requires motor learning to get the movement down correctly.

The kettlebell will be hiked between the legs.

The explosive hip drive, which is the same as the kettlebell swing, will project the kettlebell vertically and close to your body so that the kettlebell lands in the rack position.

There should be no banging with the kettlebell on the outside of the forearm, but the kettlebell should land safely and be positioned securely on the outside of the arm.

STEP 3

In lowering the kettlebell, the clean movement is reversed. The kettlebell is now hiked down and back into the start position between your legs in preparation for the next rep.

The entire movement sequence is then repeated to continue with repetitions of the clean.

I'll be up front with you: the clean can be tricky to learn.

It may be one of the more challenging exercises to get a feel for and learn the proper motor control and timing.

However, with continued practice and establishing a strong explosive hip drive, the kettlebell clean can be learned by anyone and is an effective stand-alone exercise or as a key component of a kettlebell complex.

Remember, it's critical to have the kettlebell swing technique down before attempting the clean or the snatch.

THE SNATCH

The kettlebell snatch is the kingpin of kettlebell exercises.

It's a highly explosive movement and an expressive display of dynamic power, strength, and ultimate conditioning.

The truth is that after the swing has been learned and the movement programmed effectively, the snatch is easy to figure out.

Use the explosive hip drive to project the kettlebell overhead.

The kettlebell snatch is essentially the same movement of the one-hand kettlebell swing only you are finishing with the bell overhead. This requires much more total-body energy.

THE PATH OF THE KETTLEBELL

Let's talk about the path of the kettlebell snatch.

We've talked about how the one-hand kettlebell swing projects the kettlebell horizontally.

Well, the kettlebell clean brings the kettlebell closer to your body and up your body.

The kettlebell snatch path is somewhere in the middle of the swing and the clean. The path is closer to your body than a one-hand swing, but it's not as close as a kettlebell clean.

The key to the exercise is the explosive hip drive and the breathing. Utilize biomechanical matched breathing, which applies to the swing and clean as well.

The exhalation matches the force production.

When the kettlebell is elevated overhead, the exhalation will be with the forward kettlebell movement or explosive hip drive.

As the kettlebell goes overhead, the kettlebell will be positioned on the forearm, as with the clean, and there is no banging. It is a small punch of the wrist at the top that allows the kettlebell to be positioned safely on the forearm without any banging as the kettlebell goes overhead and is repositioned.

The kettlebell should not be flipping or banging at all. If this happens, you will need to spend more time learning the correct motor skill. This requires practice and proper instruction.

Once it's learned, it should become automatic – that's the goal of learning any motor skill.

As the kettlebell reaches approximately eye-level height, this is where you will start to reposition the kettlebell so it is positioned safely on the forearm at the top of the lockout position.

The kettlebell snatch is an explosive expression of human body movement, ultimate conditioning, and high level of strength and power. This is the highest level of the kettlebell ballistic exercises since it takes the kettlebell through an extreme range of motion.

The bell goes from being positioned in the hike position during the hip hinge to being elevated overhead in one quick, explosive movement.

Here are the keys to the snatch:

- The same principles as the swing apply to the snatch.
- Snatch the kettlebell from the hike position to a full elbow lockout overhead in one smooth, explosive movement.
- The kettlebell MUST be caught properly at the top of the snatch without banging on the forearm.
- The upper arm is parallel to the head at the top position.
- The lowering of the kettlebell from the top is a controlled drop, returning to the hike position to prepare for the next snatch rep.
- Hip explosiveness and biomechanical breathing must occur to maximize power production.

THE KETTLEBELL PRESS

The next exercise is also known as the strict press or the military press.

The biggest misunderstanding about this exercise is that most people think it's just a shoulder exercise. It's actually another full body exercise because it requires full muscular tension through your trunk and abdominals.

You're also using the glutes, the quads, and firmly rooting your feet into the ground so that everything is stable and secure to press the kettlebell overhead.

It's important to get strong and stable, get tight through your entire body, starting from the rack position.

One of the great things about the kettlebell press is that it can be used to improve maximal strength.

For example, many kettlebell enthusiasts have the goal of pressing half of their body weight with a kettlebell, which is considered an extremely strong kettlebell press.

First, a couple of tips with the press.

GRIP

Make sure to squeeze the kettlebell with your grip hand as hard as you can.

This helps to increase your strength and secure the bell in your hand for a powerful press.

I also like to make a fist with the opposite hand to increase total-body tension through the upper extremities. This aids stability and upper body tightness.

BREATH

There are a couple of options when it comes to breathing as you perform the kettlebell press.

You can inhale before pressing and exhale as you press the kettlebell overhead.

Or, you can inhale and hold the breath, called a Valsalva maneuver, exhaling at the top in the lockout position. Then you inhale on the way down.

These are the different breathing options that really come down to personal preference and training experience. Try both, and use the method that will give you more pressing power and strength.

THE RACK

The press starts by cleaning the kettlebell to the rack position. Get your body tight, and then press straight up overhead into a lockout position.

The upper arm should be parallel to the ear, and the elbow should be fully extended or locked out at the top of the press.

From there, you will just bring the kettlebell down, lowering the kettlebell safely into the rack position before performing another repetition.

Here's a review of the kettlebell press:

- Press from the rack position.
- Use full-body muscular tension prior to pressing.
- Maintain a good position – neutral spine, knees locked, feet planted.
- Keep a vertical forearm throughout the press – very important.
- Keep the wrist straight; do not let it hyperextend.
- Lock the elbow at the top.
- Breathe properly (biomechanical breathing).

SUMMARY

These 7 exercises are the kettlebell fundamentals, the essentials.

Whether you're a beginner or advanced, these are still the primary exercises to be developed and improved. Your foundation is built off of these exercises.

More advanced kettlebell progressions include double kettlebell exercises, different press variations including the bent press, and many other exercises and progressions that build on these fundamentals.

To check out a great training session using the fundamentals, be sure to check out **"The Skill Session"** on RdellaTraining.com with a free PDF of this workout.

http://rdellatraining.com/kettlebell-workout-the-skill-session

A FEW WORDS ABOUT DOUBLE KETTLEBELL TRAINING

Double kettlebell training is training with a pair of kettlebells and not just one.

The many benefits of double kettlebell training include:

- Improved metabolic demands
- Increased hormonal changes
- Enhanced fat loss
- Better muscle-building effects (best way to add muscle with kettlebells)

THE NEXT LEVEL IN KETTLEBELL PERFORMANCE

I thought about whether to include double kettlebell training concepts in *The Edge of Strength* but ultimately decided to exclude double kettlebell training. Because this approach is based on fundamentals, I'll save the double kettlebell exercises and programming for future writings.

But, you should know I'm a huge fan of double kettlebell work after – and only after – the single kettlebell skills have been firmly grounded.

Adding a second kettlebell will no doubt take things to the next level in this Strength Stack. Maybe that could be called Strength Stack #3b.

With advanced exercises, it's critical to have a rock solid base with the fundamentals, specifically the movement patterns of the exercises mentioned in this chapter.

CHAPTER 23: POWERLIFTING ISN'T JUST FOR POWERLIFTERS

"Hard and simple are the keys to big and strong."
-Mark Rippetoe

STRENGTH STACK #4

The barbell is the king of strength. It's the tool that makes you feel instantly powerful and strong.

Soon after discovering kettlebells, I got back into barbell training, but with one big difference.

I started to learn what the hell I was doing.

After that a weekend-long workshop led by Pavel Tsatsouline, I knew I was back with the barbell – this time for life and with purpose.

I started applying the movement and biomechanical principles to the barbell with the basic power lifts: the back squat, bench press, and deadlift.

It made a big difference in my training and results, much greater than anything I had ever experienced in the past. I got stronger, started moving better, and actually felt like I knew exactly what I was doing with the barbell.

When I started training so many years ago, I never received the necessary instruction with any of these lifts.

For the bench press, the only coaching I ever got was to get on the bench, grab the bar, and then press the weight off your chest. And, that's exactly what I did for many years.

That was the bodybuilding bench press that many of us gym rats did back then.

Coaching – what coaching?

The most important thing I can tell you right now is that the bench press and all the power lifts are technical.

Just like kettlebells and even bodyweight training, **the power lifts require technical proficiency** and basic knowledge about how to use the tool properly for the squat, press, and deadlift.

The power lifts are hugely beneficial for all of us, not just powerlifters.

Barbell training is the best method for maximum strength development simply because we can load the bar to maximum loads.

Kettlebells will definitely get you strong, but barbells will help you get stronger. There's no strength coach I know that would even debate that point.

First, let's define general "barbell training" because the term is actually very broad. When someone says barbell training, what exactly do they mean?

THE 3 AREAS OF BARBELL TRAINING

BASIC BARBELL TRAINING (BBT)

These exercises are used for bodybuilding, general strength development, and accessory lifting exercises.

This area could also be called weight training, which is different from weightlifting.

Examples of basic lifts and exercises are biceps curls, good mornings, front squats, barbell rows, shrugs, close-grip bench presses, and many other exercises.

POWERLIFTING (PL)

These consist of 3 contested lifts:

- **Deadlift**
- **Back squat**
- **Bench press**

Even though the **standing barbell military press** is NOT a power lift, I include it in the big lifts. But it is not considered true powerlifting. Since many people may not be able to or desire to bench, the standing military press is a great alternative.

The world would be a much stronger place if everyone deadlifted, squatted, and pressed. If we did nothing else, we would be a planet full of strong and powerful people.

I'll be doing these lifts for as long as I am physically able.

OLYMPIC LIFTING (OL)

Olympic weightlifting or Olympic lifting consists of only 2 contested lifts:

- **Snatch**
- **Clean and jerk**

If you compete in weightlifting, you are a truly a specialist in these exercises.

This doesn't mean they are only for those who choose to compete in the sport of Olympic weightlifting.

This chapter offers an overview of the barbell fundamentals and will focus on the power lifts.

We'll cover OL in the next chapter in Strength Stack #5.

WHY ISN'T POWERLIFTING STACK #5?

Powerlifting is developing maximum (or limit) strength, so why isn't this the top strength stack?

These progressions are based on technical proficiency, and while PL is technical, there is nothing that demands the fast movement with maximal loads as required in the Olympic lifts.

Barbell training, whether you perform PL or OL, is an incredible tool.

You've got 2 options for barbell training.

Join a gym or invest in the equipment.

If you go the gym route, it's important to find a gym that allows chalk and has a good barbell set-up.

The "chalk test" is a great way to identify a good strength gym. If the gym doesn't allow the use of chalk – find a real strength-training gym. You can also search "local barbell club" online to see what you come up with, or check in with powerliftingwatch.com to locate a gym in your area.

If you have a home gym set-up, then maybe barbells are the next investment to add. Of course, an initial barbell set up is a financial investment. It's an investment that pays, if you're going to use them.

You could start off with an initial set up for a few hundred bucks or much more, depending on the poundage and what you get.

A few hundred bucks for the lifetime benefits I've discussed in this book is not much of an investment at all, and there is no better investment than in yourself.

For a home gym, here's what I would recommend for basic barbell training.

- A decent quality bar
- Plates
- Collars

- Rubber matt
- Power rack or squat rack

This is not for Olympic weightlifting, as OL will require bumper plates, a platform or proper flooring, and higher quality bars for the bar turnover needed in faster, more explosive lifts.

If you're new to barbells, a general recommendation for plate totals to start with for males is around 300 pounds, for females around 150 pounds.

THE LIFTS

These 4 exercises I've mentioned are some of the most effective full-body strength exercises we have available to us.

Are they easy?

Of course not.

This is one reason why most people don't do them.

But, the results will last a lifetime.

There is no person that wouldn't benefit from these lifts.

These exercises are fitness minimalism to produce superior results. I'm not saying everybody needs to perform max attempt lifts. The lifts, in general, are extremely beneficial for everyone.

The squat and the deadlift are exercises that should be for a lifetime. Let's talk about these lifts and the value of each.

Before we go any further, I want you to suspend any preconceived notions you have about powerlifting.

THE BARBELL SQUAT

The squat is also one of the most debated exercises in the fitness industry due to technique variations and differences in squat patterns.

The squat requires great technique and incredible strength throughout the entire body. There's nothing we are not using when performing a heavy barbell squat.

As with many exercises in *The Edge of Strength*, the squat is not just a leg exercise. It's a full-body exercise.

The squat has many variations. For simplicity I'm going to only address the back squat, which is the competitive squat in powerlifting.

Here are key technical points to remember in the barbell back squat.

THE SET-UP

Make sure that when you approach the bar you get set properly before un-racking the bar. We'll discuss proper set-up below.

It's always all about the set-up, and this will be a recurring theme as we cover other lifts.

Low bar or high bar? Well, it depends. For PL style, the low bar position is mostly advocated. For OL, the high bar position is preferred due to mimicking the demands of the Olympic lifts.

HAND PLACEMENT

Hand placement is important, and if you can place your hands closer to each other on the bar, it makes for a tighter set-up in regards to the upper body.

By bringing your hands closer together on the bar, it helps to stabilize the upper body and makes for a tighter, more efficient lift.

BREATHING

Breathing is extremely important once you load the bar and when you step back and get ready to squat.

You want to take a deep breath with the diaphragmatic breathing technique discussed earlier in Chapter 6 – Move Well.

This will significantly improve performance and trunk stability to keep your back strong and stable as you descend and ascend in the squat.

Again, take a deep breath, and hold it throughout a full repetition. Exhale at the top.

This makes a rigid cylinder or tight column of your trunk musculature so it can effectively stabilize and support heavier loads.

FOOT PLACEMENT

Make sure your feet are set before you squat.

Foot stance will vary depending on technique and body structure, but in general take about shoulder-width stance or slightly wider.

This goes back to the set-up. Make sure your feet are in the right position and are stable before you squat.

Take the time to properly prepare before you go through the lifr.

THE GLUTES

Something that's not always talked about is using the glutes prior to the squat. Here's what you want to do.

When you step back away from the rack, make sure to squeeze the glutes tight to stabilize your spine and pelvis for maximal stability prior to descending.

Again, squeeze the glutes and squeeze them hard prior to performing the squat. This is an important point because it improves safety and stabilty.

BACK POSITION

Keep the spine in neutral or slight extension throughout the squat.

The previous steps we talked about will help us to keep a stable spine.

What we want to avoid is a rounding of the back or forward flexion as this places great demand on the intervertebral disks, thus increasing the potential risk for injury.

Neutral spine or slight extension is the key. Think about staying tall (or chest up) to keep the spine in optimal position. This is a point I feel strongly about, so if you remember one thing here – remember this.

KNEE POSITION

Keep the knees in line with the toes or even slightly outside to minimize stress on your joints and maximize torque in the hips.

The "knees out" cue is often used to prevent the inward (or valgus) knee collapse, although use caution with this tip so as not to excessively drive the knees outward, which can be very uncomfortable especially as the poundages increase.

Another cue to think about to effectively stabilize the hips, knees, and feet is to *screw your feet into the ground*. Much like the breathing techniques to stabilize the spine, this cue helps to stabilize the lower extremities.

Break parallel, and squat deep. Breaking parallel means the hips are below the knees at the bottom position. There's a saying that if you can't go below parallel, the weight is too heavy.

There's no data to support that squatting deep is a bad for normal, healthy knees, and the data is actually supportive for joint health.

A deeper squat is more functional, builds more strength, and maintains full range of motion in the knee structures when done properly.

Explode Up from the Squat

Once you've lowered past parallel, explode up out of the hole. The hole is the bottom position of the squat.

When you squat down, shift towards accelerating the bar up through the top of the lift.

THE DEADLIFT

The deadlift is the most accessible and fundamental of the power lifts. It's a simple exercise, yet it is also very complex to perform correctly.

The barbell deadlift is full-body strength and works virtually every major muscle group in your body.

Picking up a loaded barbell from the floor is a wonderful expression of full-body strength that's difficult for any other exercise to match. The deadlift will benefit any human for a lifetime, and even 80+ year olds continue to benefit from the lift.

The deadlift is available to almost all humans as a way to improve total-body functional strength like nothing else.

A heavy deadlift is extremely demanding and taxing on our nervous system and requires proper technique, programming, and certainly recovery between training sessions.

There are different techniques (e.g., sumo and conventional) and different implements (e.g., kettlebell, dumbbell, barbell, and odd objects) to perform a deadlift.

The barbell deadlift is the best way to develop total-body strength because we can load the bar to maximal loads.

Just as a review, the **conventional deadlift** is when the arms are placed on the outside of the legs. For many people, the conventional deadlift is the most common way to deadlift.

The **sumo deadlift** is when the arms are on the inside of the legs. The legs are positioned in a wider stance.

There are benefits and limitations of each.

Ultimately, I believe which deadlift style you choose comes down to personal preference, and certainly you can make the case towards body types and advantages with the different styles.

Train both for a reasonable amount of time (one to three months), and find the one that suits you the best.

The conventional deadlift is the most common, so I'll cover the key technical considerations of that variation.

THE SET-UP

As with the squat and other lifts, you probably know by now that the deadlift is all about the set-up. Take your time in getting set as you approach the bar, and be sure to consider the following points.

The more you focus on set-up, the more automatic it will become so that you're not thinking about too many things. Instead you just do them automatically, which is the value of practice.

THE STANCE

The stance is approximately shoulder-width apart in the conventional deadlift. (As mentioned, a wider stance is used for sumo-style deadlifts).

KEEP THE BAR CLOSE

The bar needs to be close to the body, essentially touching the shin or over the midfoot. If the bar is positioned away from the body, that's an inefficient set-up prior to deadlifting the bar.

Bar position is critical. Keep the bar place close to the body at your set-up and also throughout the entire pull.

Think **"vertical bar path"** in the deadlift as you keep the bar close to your body.

THE GRIP

Your grip will be just outside of your legs and not too wide (conventional).

The alternating grip is most commonly used, where one hand is pronated (palm down) and one hand is supinated (palm up).

To avoid developing significant asymmetry here, it is recommended to alternate the grip with training sets, although you will likely find that one position is stronger or more comfortable than the other as the load increases.

THE HIPS

Typically the hips are positioned higher than the knees, but lower than the shoulders.

This position is ideal for most people to keep the body in a good position and **maximize leg drive** to lift the bar from the floor.

APPLICATION OF TENSION

Once you grip the bar in your set-up and get in the proper position to prepare for the pull, the application of muscular tension is extremely important.

Before you initiate the pull of the bar off of the ground, make sure that you get tight and stable throughout your body. Here's what to do prior to lifting the bar:

- Tighten your shoulders by gripping the bar
- Engage your lats

- Tighten the glutes, quads, and hams by screwing your feet into the ground
- Take a deep breath
- Make sure that the back is in neutral or preferably slight extension – think "chest up"

Once your body is completely tight and stable using full body muscular tension, you are ready for a safe and efficient deadlift.

This may be one of the most important points for a safe and strong deadlift, so please remember to use full-body muscular tension prior to initiating the bar from the floor.

DRIVE THROUGH YOUR FEET

When you initiate the pull from the floor, drive your feet down through the ground instead of pulling the bar up. Think "push, not pull."

This simple cue will help you to drive leg strength and power to get heavy loads up from the ground.

SET YOUR BACK

To minimize risk for injury, this step is important. Many people perform an unsafe deadlift by rounding the back to initiate the deadlift.

This big mistake greatly increases the risk for injury because of the increase in spinal loading to the intervertebral discs.

Rounding the back or forward flexing places extreme stress on the posterior aspect of the lumbar disc. This means it's easier to herniate or rupture the intervertebral disc.

I'm speaking from personal experience because this is precisely how I was injured so many years ago.

To minimize this stress and pressure on the disc space, start with and maintain a slight lumbar and thoracic extension. Injuries will be greatly reduced if this key technique is implemented.

If you remember only one thing about deadlifts, **remember to keep the spine locked in neutral or slight extension.**

THE BENCH PRESS

The bench press is an exercise that gets a bad rap these days. But is there any more powerful upper body developer than the bench press? I don't think so.

After learning how to properly perform the bench press after so many years of inattention to technique, I can tell you that it is a very effective total-body strength builder and is safe when proper technique is executed.

GRIP WIDTH

Grip width is individual, but a couple of key considerations are to keep the bar over the wrist and keep the wrist over your elbow.

This means that the forearm is vertical and allows for an optimal position for pressing power.

I much prefer and strongly recommend a full-thumb grip (as opposed to a thumbless grip) for bar security. Wrap the thumb around the bar and train safe.

THE SET-UP

Grip the bar hard, and squeeze your shoulder blades together to set and stabilize the upper body.

The glutes remain in contact with the bench, and the back is arched.

SQUEEZE THE GLUTES

Squeeze your glutes and drive your heels down through the floor, which promotes full-body tension and a tight set-up.

ENGAGE THE LATS

The lats are key in a strong press. Think about "breaking or bending the bar" as you set up which will fire the lats.

If you hold the bar and imagine you are bending or breaking it, the lats automatically turn on, so this is a simple but valuable tip.

USE THE LEGS

The use of the legs is often missed, but it is very effective in improving press strength and allowing you to use full-body tension for a stronger press.

A simple cue is to think about extending the legs as you drive your feet through the floor.

THINK FULL BODY

Think about using your full body in the bench press, not just your pecs and arms.

By thinking about using your entire body during the lift, you'll add strength, safety, and effectiveness to the bench press.

LOCKOUT

Make sure to lock out or fully extend your arms when you press the bar up at the end of the rep.

Don't short-change yourself with incomplete or partial reps.

Work through the full range of motion, and lock the elbows at the end of the press.

THE MILITARY PRESS (STANDING PRESS)

The overhead barbell press is a valuable exercise. It's exceptional for full-body strength; yet many people don't perform it.

If you want to feel instantly powerful, there's nothing more satisfying than pressing a heavy weight over your head.

Here are a few key considerations to perform an effective overhead press.

GRIP

When you grab the bar in your set-up, grip the bar firmly to increase muscular tension in the arms and upper body.

Wrap your thumbs around the bar – do not use a thumbless grip. And make sure the bar is secure in your hand.

A strong, firm grip will boost your pressing power by increasing upper-body muscular tension and put you in a much more stable position from which to press.

One way to do this is to think about "breaking the bar," as mentioned to engage the lats in the bench press.

VERTICAL FOREARMS

Keep your forearms vertical as you get in position to press the bar.

This puts the bar in the rack position (where the bar sits on the anterior deltoids and at the clavicle or slightly above).

The vertical position of the forearms should place your hands approximately shoulder-width apart or just slightly outside.

The forearm position sets up for a strong overhead press in a safe, efficient plane of motion, keeping the bar close to your body as you elevate the bar to full lockout overhead.

It's very important to set up and maintain vertical forearm position for an effective press.

FULL-BODY TENSION

As with the grip, this will help to increase upper-body tension. Think about keeping tight from your feet all the way up through the rest of your body.

Plant your feet firmly on the ground, and think about screwing your feet into floor.

Keep the feet about shoulder-width apart, and keep the feet pointing straight ahead or with a slight toe-out position. This will increase the tension in your lower body for strength and stability.

Also, keep your glutes tight and abs tense before your press.

Basically, everything in your body – from your feet, through your hips and spine, and up to your shoulders and grip –should be tight before you press.

This full-body tension applied will be critical to a strong, stable overhead press. There's a saying about the press: *"You can't shoot a cannon from a canoe."*

BREATH

If you're an experienced lifter, take a breath and hold it for the ascent of the barbell press.

Once overhead, let your breath out, and inhale on the way down. Alternatively, you may take a breath at the top to stabilize and hold your breath again as you lower the bar to the start position.

Holding your breath (or Valsalva maneuver) is important for a safe, strong press.

If you're a novice, you should definitely consider a slightly different approach to breathing until you're accustomed to the Valsalva.

Take a deep breath, and exhale as you drive the bar up.

This is not a bad alternative, and it's a better breathing pattern if you're not used to the holding technique of the Valsalva. Recent data supports that the Valsalva is a more appropriate technique for the experienced lifter, as compared to the novice.

Proper breathing is power, I hope this point is clear by now. (If not, revisit Chapter 6 – Move Well.)

BAR POSITION AT THE TOP

As the bar is elevated overhead, the finish position is with arms fully locked out overhead. The bar should be positioned directly over your shoulder joints (the glenohumeral joints).

If observing someone press from the side view, the bar should be directly over the shoulder joints. Look for a vertical line from the middle of the foot, through the shoulders, and up to the bar overhead with the arms fully extended.

Common faults would be to finish with the bar positioned more anteriorly (too far to the front) or not completing a full lockout of the elbows.

This overhead position allows for great shoulder and thoracic mobility, as well as superior strength with a heavy load.

As with the deadlift, keep the bar close to your body as you are pressing. You don't want to bar move away from your body as you complete the motion.

The vertical forearm position will keep the bar close to your body for an efficient bar path on the drive up (and back down).

For an extremely comprehensive understanding of these lifts, I'd definitely recommend checking out *Starting Strength* by Mark Rippetoe.

CHAPTER 24: OLYMPIC WEIGHTLIFTING

"There is literally no other sport that challenges
your strength, skill, and mental powers more fully than weightlifting."
–Arthur Dreschler

STRENGTH STACK #5: THE PINNACLE

If there's one thing I wished I had started earlier, it would be Olympic weightlifting.

I openly admit to sucking at Olympic weightlifting when I started. I know this because I still have some of my initial training videos from one of the earlier workshops I attended. Yes, there's evidence that it was bad.

But, because I stayed with these lifts and was determined to improve my skills and techniques with the lifts, they eventually got better.

Hard work and perseverance always pay off.

Perfection is not attainable, but if we
chase perfection we can chase excellence.
–Vince Lombardi

There's really nothing like performing a well-executed barbell snatch or barbell clean and jerk. Getting to that point is well worth the effort.

The clean and jerk is the exercise that demands the highest level of energy expenditure, according to the work of Verkhoshanky and Siff.

I want you to **suspend your disbelief** about Olympic weightlifting as you read this chapter.

Make sure to read through this, even if you think Olympic weightlifting isn't for you.

Weightlifting is amazing. It's one of the most amazing displays of human movement, performance, and explosive strength.

And, I don't want you to miss out.

OLYMPIC WEIGHTLIFTING BACKGROUND

One chapter on this subject is an almost an impossibility.

Keep in mind this is only an overview and hopefully enough to whet your appetite or, if you're a weightlifter, give you a few new insights.

This is simply an introduction and basic background on the ultimate expression of human performance: Olympic lifting, or OL as I'll refer to it moving forward.

There are many excellent books on this subject that I can recommend to you:

- Greg Everett's *Olympic Weightlifting*
- Greg Everett's *Olympic Weightlifting for Sports* (the more condensed version of Greg's work)
- Arthur Dreschler's *Weightlifting Encyclopedia*
- The spectacular work by Tommy Kono, *Championship Weightlifting* and *Weightlifting Olympic Style*

Olympic lifting (OL) is generally considered a strength specialist sport or can be applied as an approach to overall strength and conditioning or functional fitness approach.

The Olympic lifts consist of these 2 exercises:

- **The Snatch**
- **The Clean and Jerk**

Although there are numerous assistance exercises in OL to assist with these, the snatch and the clean and jerk are the two competitive lifts.

Both lifts are very physically demanding and require the highest level of technical proficiency, explosive strength, power, grit, and determination.

This is why, in my opinion, **OL is the pinnacle of performance.**

To do well with OL, you have to immerse yourself in these skills and get with a great coach – that's the bottom line.

If your goals are to compete, then your goal is to become a strength specialist with these lifts.

Out of all the methods I have presented in this book, OL is by far the most technically demanding and can require the longest time to learn.

However, everyone is different, and some may pick up the skills faster than others. I happen to be one of those who required a lot of practice, hard work, and time.

Here's why I'm committed to them.

They are skills that can provide benefit for a lifetime.

I've been extremely honored to work with and learn directly from such accomplished OL coaches as Glenn Pendlay, Greg Everett, and Danny Camargo.

I've been fortunate to have the opportunity to interview many outstanding coaches and authors for **The Rdella Training® Podcast.** One of them was Matt Foreman.

In our interview, here's something that Matt said he learned from an orthopedic surgeon about the particular topic of joint health and weightlifting:

> *"A lot of people think that weightlifting is*
> *bad for your knees. It's actually the opposite.*
> *Lifting weights is one of the best things for your knees.*
> *The things that are bad for your knees are all the*
> *jump, twist, and pivot types of movements*
> *with rotational torque."*

Let's understand something that's very unique to this strength skill.

As I mentioned, OL can last a lifetime. It's a sport that really has no barriers, if you think about it. Competition age ranges are from u-13 to 80+. The only limitation in OL is your decision not to engage.

Yes, there can be real physical limitations or restrictions which prevent you from participating, but assuming good movement and mobility are present, there are no limitations other than your beliefs.

Of course, the use of OL should be carefully considered before initiating them. As we covered earlier, never do something because someone says so or you think it looks cool or whatever. Do something because you have clarity about your reason why and understand how it fits into your specific goals and long-term approach.

With the rise of CrossFit, OL has had a major resurgence, which is fantastic for fitness. CrossFit utilizes OL by performing high reps that are done for a specific time. However, many top coaches will openly state that this is not the way to perform such highly skilled and technically demanding lifts.

There are safety concerns to keep in mind, as with any physical activity, but we all have to make our own decisions about how we train and why. Safety is always going to be my #1 training priority. Remember that "safe strength" is key to becoming bulletproof.

I want to encourage and inspire you to get involved in weightlifting; however, it's important to be transparent regarding when and where it should be used.

Like every other strength training method, it <u>must</u> be a match for your training goals.

THE BIG CHALLENGE

The major challenge with OL is learning the technical proficiency to perform the lifts correctly.

Olympic weightlifting is a high-skill strength movement, if not the highest, so it requires great coaching to learn the movements with the right technique to maximize performance and minimize risk for injury.

It requires technique on top of a prerequisite baseline of movement, mobility, and stability. That's why it's Stack #5.

My experience with OL is relegated to only the last few years, and I have immersed myself in it due to the challenge, the technical demands, the skill of movement, and the explosive strength benefits. When I do something, I go "all in" and that's what I have done with OL.

Frankly, I love it.

There's nothing more exciting, challenging, and rewarding than explosively lifting a barbell overhead in a dynamic and fluid movement.

Will OL contribute to aesthetic goals?

Absolutely, but this is not why you perform Olympic weightlifting.

Be in it for the challenge and the path it will lead you down, not just in terms of physical strength, but also mental preparation, attention to detail, and long-term training.

WHY OLYMPIC WEIGHTLIFTING?

You perform them to get better at the skill, to improve the performance qualities, conquer the challenges, test your limits, and to enjoy the beautiful movement and the sport.

Anyone looking to advance their physical strength performance skills should consider training the Olympic lifts.

Anyone interested in improving mobility, stability, motor control and coordination, explosive strength, and athleticism should think about training with OL.

Even if you don't have aspirations of competing, that doesn't mean you should exclude yourself from learning OL.

But, only do it because it makes sense for you and will help you achieve the things you want. If OL can help you on the path to becoming the best version of yourself, then do it. It's as simple as that.

Here are some of the main benefits of OL to consider:

- Improve total body strength
- Increase explosive strength and power development
- Improve motor skill improvement and coordination
- Improve functional hypertrophy
- Improve mobility and stability
- Enhance athleticism
- Improve mental power
- Increase flexibility
- Continuous development of motor and strength skills
- Competition opportunities
- Enhance sport performance
- Conquer new challenges

I could keep going as the benefits of OL are many. But let's move onto training so you can discover them for yourself.

3 STEPS FOR PROGRESSION WITH OL

1 – COMMIT TO THE LIFTS

I believe the 1st critical step in weightlifting (or any strength-training method) is your commitment.

COMMIT TO THESE LIFTS FOR A MINIMUM OF 1 YEAR.

Understand it may be a challenge, but you are going to commit yourself to the process of learning how to perform the Olympic lifts – no matter how long it may take or what you have to sacrifice.

The rewards will be worth it.

2 – LEARN ALL YOU CAN

I always recommend fully reading about and learning the basics of something before getting started (whether that's kettlebells, barbells, or anything else).

You'll understand a training method on a deeper level, ensuring you aren't just going through the motions.

With that said, get the book, *Olympic Weightlifting* by Greg Everett. This is essential reading for learning all about the sport of OL, and it offers a thorough overview that contains everything you need to know.

And, if you have experience – find other ways to keep learning and keep growing.

These are skills to develop for a lifetime.

3 – FIND A COACH OR CLUB

Although this can be the challenging part, try to find a qualified coach. This is a very important step that will accelerate your progress.

Finding a qualified coach takes due diligence on your part.

It takes effort and research to search for a good coach, but it's worth every ounce of energy because it will accelerate your progress and results faster than anything else.

If you're in the United States, you can go to:

www.teamusa.org/USA-Weightlifting

What if you don't have a local coach?

I hear this question a lot.

Online coaching is better than no coaching. And, this applies whether you're new or advanced and applies to any method in this book.

Online coaching is not ideal for OL because it requires a lot of effort on the student and coach, but it's better than no coaching at all.

In addition to your coach, make sure to get around the right people. If you're more advanced, surround yourself with other great lifters. Train around the people who will make you better.

Google "local barbell club" or "local weightlifting club" to see what's in your area.

OL PROGRAMMING

"The biggest separator with people who do well and those who don't is that the people who do well don't quit."
–Coach Glenn Pendlay

Weightlifting is hard.

That's why this is the top tier progression in Strength Stacking.

For some of you, it may come easier, but for most, it's very challenging. Luckily, there are many great OL programs available to us.

The main thing with the simple program I'll outline or any program is to pick one and stick to it.

There's nothing magical or complex about this program.

It's based on the fundamentals of the snatch and clean and jerk.

And, just like the proven 5 x 5 or 3 x 3 programs, this is effective.

The best programs are the simple programs. The following program template is a variation that comes directly from my experience with renowned Olympic weightlifting coach Glenn Pendlay.

My understanding from Coach Pendlay is that he prefers the simple programs that are built around the fundamentals. Assistance exercises are useful and valuable to improve technique and skill, but remember they are done to "assist" the primary lifts.

If you're searching for a weightlifting program, keep things simple, fundamental, and make sure it addresses your top goals.

The primary lifts are the focus of your training.

Basic Program Concepts:

- This is a 5-day training template
- Most training days, work sets are for 10 total reps for each of the lifts

BASIC OL PROGRAM TEMPLATE:

To get better with the Olympic lifts, you have to practice the skills of Olympic lifting. That means you snatch a lot and clean and jerk a lot.

This program is immersed in the lifts, but will vary the intensity and reps each training session.

It's a short program for only a few weeks. I've used this program as a quick **2–4 week training cycle.**

	Mon	Tues	Wed	Fri	Sat
Snatch	2 x 5	5 – 3 – 1	3 x 3	5 x 2	6 x 1
Clean & Jerk	2 x 5	5 – 3 – 1	3 x 3	5 x 2	6 x 1
Front Squat	2 x 5	5 – 3 – 1	3 x 3	5 x 2	6 x 1

Sets with lower reps are higher intensity and vice versa.

This is a low-volume but focused program that I always benefit from. It's important to moderate the intensities.

The Saturday session with "singles" is the heavy day, but it really goes according to how you feel.

A BRIEF OVERVIEW OF TECHNICAL ASPECTS OF EXERCISES

THE SNATCH

The snatch is the most technical and demands a high level of mobility, stability, flexibility, and strength.

The bar is gripped from the floor and taken overhead with one explosive movement, consisting of 3 pulls (see below).

Here's the exercise description of the snatch:

As usual, **the set-up is key.**

- Set a snatch-width grip. This is when the hands are wide enough that the bar contacts the body in the crease of the hips when standing tall with the bar at arms' length.
- The feet are approximately hip-width apart and toes turned out slightly with the weight balanced evenly.
- The knees are pushed out.
- The back is arched in slight extension.
- The arms are straight and elbows turned out to the sides.
- The head and eyes are forward.
- To begin the lift, drive with the legs against the floor (1st pull) with the hips and shoulder rising simultaneously until the bar is at approximately mid-thigh.
- Aggressively push against the floor, and extend the hips explosively. (2nd pull)
- Keep the bar close to the body, allowing it to contact the hips as they reach extension (*Bar contact is important, but you are not smacking the hips with the bar)
- Once you have fully extended your body, jump the feet outward. Move into your squat stance as you pull your elbows up and to the sides.
- As the bar is vertically elevating, begin to pull yourself down into a squat under the bar. (3rd pull)
- Continue actively bringing the bar into the overhead position as you pull down into the squat.
- Stabilize the bar overhead.
- Stand up while keeping the bar positioned overhead.
- Once you've stood completely with the bar in control, safely return the bar to the floor.

THE CLEAN

The clean is the first part of the clean and jerk, and it can be used independently.

In this move, the athlete takes the bar from the floor to the shoulders.

The **power clean** is another variation, and it's commonly believed to be easier to learn.

The power clean essentially finishes in a quarter squat position (as opposed to full squat in the clean), so you are receiving the bar higher in the power clean.

Again, the difference between the clean and power clean is the height of the receiving position of the barbell. The same can be said about the snatch and **power snatch.**

Here are the key points in the clean:

- Set up correctly:
- Get set with a clean-width grip, positioning the hands slightly outside shoulder-width.
- The feet are approximately hip-width and toes turned slightly outward.
- The weight is balanced evenly and knees are pushed out.
- The back is arched completely.
- The arms are straight and elbows turned out to the sides.
- Head and eyes are forward.
- To begin, drive with the legs against the floor to stand, and simultaneously raise the hips and shoulders until the bar is at approximately mid-thigh. (1st pull)
- Continue to aggressively push against the floor as you extend the hips explosively, keeping the bar close to the body and allowing it to contact the upper thighs as the hips move into extension (2nd pull)
- Once extended, slightly jump the feet out into the receiving stance as you aggressively pull your elbows up and to the sides.
- As the bar is being pulled upward, pull yourself down into a squat under the bar to prepare to receive the clean. (3rd pull)
- Bring the elbows around the bar quickly and into the "rack" position as you descend into the squat.
- Use the "rebound" effect in the bottom of the squat to help stand up as quickly as possible.
- Once you stand up completely with the bar in control, return it to the floor (or continue to the next part – the jerk).

THE JERK (SPLIT JERK)

This is the second part of the clean and jerk.

The clean and jerk is the most physically demanding exercise in terms of energy expenditure.

When compared to other related exercises, the clean and jerk produced the highest absolute energy expenditure across lifters, according to the work by Siff.

The jerk is a controlled dip, powerful drive, and then re-dip (catch) under the bar. The split jerk, which we'll look at now, is dynamic and explosive. It is the competitive style jerk.

Let's review the keys to the jerk:

- Make sure the bar is secure in the jerk "rack position."
- Set-up correctly:
- The feet are approximately hip-width apart and toes slightly turned out.
- Keep the weight balanced on the heels while maintaining full foot contact with the floor.
- Be sure to take a stabilizing breath before initiating the jerk.
- To initiate the jerk, bend slightly at the knees, and keep a vertical torso with the weight on the heels.
- Transition immediately at the bottom of this dip to drive explosively with the legs against the floor to accelerate the barbell upward.
- When the extension of the legs is complete, quickly begin pushing against the bar with the arms and lifting the feet to transition into the split position.
- Finish with the arms into a locked-out overhead position.
- Secure and stabilize the bar overhead before recovering from the split into a standing position with the bar still overhead.
- Step back with the front leg, then step forward with the back leg when returning to the standing position.
- Return the bar to the floor safely.

The snatch and the clean and jerk are outstanding exercises that can benefit many people besides athletes.

Again, a challenge is learning these lifts correctly and nailing every step listed here. You can see why OL is a skill that definitely requires coaching.

KEY ASSISTANCE EXERCISES FOR WEIGHTLIFTING

There are **countless assistance exercises** for the Olympic lifts. The key is to select the ones that are most important to you and will help you the most.

Here are a few that are extremely valuable.

FRONT SQUATS

The front squat is extremely common with OL because it so closely assists in the strength and power for the lifts.

The front squat is done with an upright torso and the bar in the front rack position.

This lift is key to leg strength development.

Even though the front squat by itself is not a primary weightlifting exercise, it is considered mandatory with OL training.

PULLS

Pulls (clean pulls and snatch pulls) are easier to learn and help promote triple extension (hip, knee, and ankle) with the lifts.

SNATCH BALANCE

The snatch balance is an excellent exercise to improve overhead strength, stability, and confidence for the snatch.

PUSH PRESS

The push press is valuable to develop upper-body strength and explosive leg power.

The push press is also an important progression in learning the jerk.

ROMANIAN DEADLIFTS

Romanian deadlifts (RDLs) have been very useful for athletes to develop the back arch, as well as glute and hamstring strength.

RDLs are another commonly used assistance exercise for OL.

The training suggestions above include only a few of many valuable exercises to assist in the development of weightlifting.

FROM KETTLEBELLS TO OLYMPIC LIFTS

If you're a kettlebell enthusiast, you may be thinking it will be easy to learn OL.

I want to be honest with you: it's a hard transition.

In my experience, the hip power production and neuromuscular learning is entirely different going from kettlebell training to OL.

Kettlebells are easier to learn in terms of hip power (e.g., the swing) as compared to weightlifting, where the hip angle is much smaller and the bar path is much more vertical.

It's an entirely different neuromuscular process.

This is something to be aware of and another reason why Olympic weightlifting is the pinnacle of performance – Strength Stack #5.

OL is lifting explosively with maximum loads – there's nothing like it.

This chapter was simply a brief introduction to the benefits of OL. Just for perspective, *The Weightlifting Encyclopedia* is over 550 pages, all covering the techniques of OL.

It's a big topic.

I'd encourage you to check out the resources I've previously listed in this chapter and also at the end of the book.

Next, let's discuss the important topic of conditioning.

CHAPTER 25: THE IMPORTANCE OF CONDITIONING

"The best conditioning program is the one
that meets your specific needs."
–Joel Jamison

Strength and conditioning are extremely interdependent of each other and closely related, especially when we're discussing optimal human performance.

This is a book about strength.

And, you now have a great understanding about the health and performance benefits of strength and what it means to you.

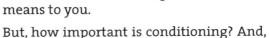

But, how important is conditioning? And, what exactly is it?

Depending on the sport or individual need, conditioning could be considered king.

Of course, the same can be said for strength or speed – it all depends on your goals.

What's most important to you . . .

STRENGTH

SPEED or

CONDITIONING?

Regardless of what ultimate skill or quality you're training for, conditioning is extremely important for most athletes and fitness enthusiasts. It may even be emphasized over strength.

Let's start by getting a working definition of what conditioning means.

Conditioning is an extremely general term. As a matter of fact, I had a hard time finding an accurate definition to use in this book.

In general, most of us associate conditioning with aerobic power and cardiovascular fitness.

But, it's more than that.

It's a combination of cardiovascular development and muscular endurance.

Here's how I would define conditioning and it's important to understand because the word is so loosely used in fitness.

CONDITIONING IS THE STAMINA AND THE ABILITY TO ENDURE FATIGUE WITH REPEATED, INTENSE EXERCISE OR TRAINING.

Conditioning is also mental toughness.

It's the ability to overcome fatigue and not run out of gas.

Conditioning can address all **3 energy systems** that we discussed in Chapter 3 of the book: **the alatic system, the lactic system, and the aerobic system.**

Strength is our foundation, but it is not the only thing we need. We've covered many other important physical qualities such as endurance in earlier chapters. Remember if you increase one, you take from another.

The level of conditioning will completely depend on your training goals and the sport you're participating in.

If a really strong fighter is de-conditioned, guess what's going to happen?

He's going to get his ass kicked.

But, is it important for a competitive powerlifter to work on conditioning for preparation for a meet?

No, because it will take away from the primary goal.

Conditioning is relative to the goal.

As this book is focused on strength, I didn't want to exclude the topic and importance of incorporating conditioning into your program.

GREAT CONDITIONING METHODS

What's the best program or approach to conditioning?

The question is impossible to answer without knowing the specifics behind it.

So, let's talk specifics about some of the methods. Here are **six of my favorite ways to improve conditioning,** including what you'll gain from each one. Keep in mind, **there are many options,** but these are some of my personal favorites.

1 – SPRINTING

There's nothing as expressive or explosive as sprinting in a wide open field.

Sprinting is full-body freedom, and the movement dynamics build many qualities related to strength. Acceleration strength, speed strength, explosive strength are some of them.

And, for pure speed, acceleration, fat-burning benefits, muscle-building, and overall athleticism – sprinting is outstanding.

I prefer to sprint once or twice per week, depending on the primary training goal.

Don't overcomplicate it.

Make sure to start slow, depending on your background and current state of conditioning.

Anywhere from 6 to 10, 40 – to 50-yard sprints is a good place to start.

One thing to consider is that sprinting is technical. This means it does require proper mechanics and sprint technique to maximize the benefits.

I'd recommend doing some further reading on sprint technique to get a better understanding.

And, don't sprint all out – at least until you learn how to sprint.

Sprint at about 90% effort, leaving a little in the tank, especially when starting out.

It should feel effortless and fluid.

2 – JUMPING ROPE

Jumping rope is outstanding for conditioning, as well as trunk strength, dynamic stability, coordination, balance, and more.

And, it may be one of the best fat-loss secrets ever.

I typically use intervals when I do jump rope training.

Start off with a series of 30-second intervals, and see how many you can perform. Jump rope for 30 seconds, rest for 30 seconds and repeat.

Or, begin with a series of reps, and record the rounds you can do.

For example, shoot for 30 reps (30 jumps), and do multiple rounds. Write down how many rounds you finish.

Keep it simple, and scale it up or down based on where your conditioning is. There are many ways to use the jump rope, but no matter what you do, **get a baseline** and progress from there.

When I include jump rope training, it's usually as a finisher at the very end of a session.

3 – BURPEES

Most people hate them, but burpees are insanely effective for a high level of supreme conditioning.

I've discussed burpees as a fundamental exercise in bodyweight training, and there are many ways to use them in a program.

Joe DeSena, Founder of Spartan Race has called them the "ultimate exercise for humans."

How many burpees should we do?

Advanced athletes should be able to complete 100 burpees in 10 minutes or less.

For most of us, somewhere between 30 a day and 30 a week is reasonable, depending on goals.

4 – SLED WORK

Whether you use drag sleds or the Prowler, sled work is extremely effective for strength and conditioning.

And, it's not technical or hard to learn – you simply push or pull the sled and go.

If you want to build higher levels of conditioning, sled work is definitely a winner. A few rounds of sled work will improve multiple energy systems and is very effective for athletes and fitness enthusiasts of all levels.

Loaded carries are similar in benefits, but different than sleds. As an alternative to a push/pull sled, a loaded carry or farmer's walk can also be used as an effective conditioning method.

5 – KETTLEBELL SWINGS AND SNATCHES

For conditioning, kettlebell swings and snatches are definitely king.

Here's an example of a simple 4-week program I call "The Equalizer." It's a simple progression and good for building strength, as well as conditioning.

The specific goal is to increase strength of 5 sets of 10/10. That means that you do 10 swings on the right, then 10 on the left.

Many people have found that 5 sets of 10/10 is the **minimal effective dose** (MED) of the one-arm swing.

But, how do you effectively progress with the exercise to build strength and conditioning?

This template is a great solution.

This progression is different, in terms of frequency and progression, from what Pavel has brilliantly outlined in his great book, *Simple and Sinister*.

The specific goal of the program is to build up to a maximal kettlebell size that you can perform for 5 sets of 10 with outstanding swing technique.

Here are the program specifics:

3 sessions per week (Monday, Wednesday, Friday or similar pattern)

Each session, complete only 5 sets of 10 reps (for a total of 100 reps each side). Rest as needed between each set of 10/10.

The sessions are quick and time-efficient (a density training approach, covered at the end of this chapter, may work to shorten your time)

The program is designed to be used as only a part of your training approach. You can plug in "the equalizer" into what you are already doing, providing it does not detract from your primary training goal. Make sure "the equalizer" adds to what you're doing.

Here's the key to the program progression.

You *must* know the kettlebell size that you can use for 5 sets of 10 with outstanding technique. You need 2 different size kettlebells to perform this program.

In this example, let's assume you can do 5 sets of 10/10 with "rock solid" technique with the 24 kg kettlebell.

For the program, you will use a 24 kg kettlebell and ONE kettlebell size up, which would be a 28 kg kettlebell.

The program is front-loaded. First, use the "heavy" kettlebell, and then drop to your standard kettlebell size for the remaining sets.

Through the quick progressions, you ultimately work up to 4 sequential sessions of 5 sets of 10/10 with the heavier kettlebell.

Here's the program over a **4-week time period** (assuming all sessions are done 3 x week as outlined).

WEEK 1

Session 1, 28 kg 10/10 x 1 set, then 24 kg 10/10 x 4 sets

Session 2, REPEAT session 1

Session 3, 28 kg 10/10 x 2 sets, then 24 kg 10/10 x 3 sets

WEEK 2

Session 4, REPEAT session 3

Session 5, 28 kg 10/10 x 3 sets, then 24 kg 10/10 x 2 sets

Session 6, REPEAT session 5

WEEK 3

Session 7, 28 kg 10/10 x 4 sets, then 24 kg 10/10 x 1 set

Session 8, REPEAT session 7

Session 9, 28 kg 10/10 x 5 sets

WEEK 4

Sessions 10–12, REPEAT session 9

The last week of sessions are all 10/10 x 5 sets with the heavier kettlebell – one kettlebell size up from where you started.

The performance goal is to do 4 complete sessions with the heavier kettlebell size and outstanding one-arm swing technique.

A few things to keep in mind.

If you struggle with a session, repeat the session again next time. The idea is to maintain *outstanding* technique as you build strength.

It should feel "easy" as you progress through the sessions, providing you have good baseline conditioning and one-arm swing technique.

If you want to advance to a higher bell size after the program, repeat the program starting at session 1.

You could do this with a kettlebell that is 2 bell sizes up from your standard, but I've found that one bell size up allows you to barely notice the change. It may depend on what else you're doing with your training, but one kettlebell size up allows for a "creep" effect – meaning you creep up the weight slowly and allow the progression to come nice and easy.

Here are 2 potential modifications to the program.

If you want progress faster, if you're training 5 days per week, for example, you could do the program each day you train by following the progression. This is not how I've used it, but it could be a reasonable approach. This would move you through the progressions in just over 2 weeks (instead of 4 weeks).

If you're more advanced and want to be more aggressive, then use a bell size that is 2 bell sizes up. For example, if your 5 sets of 10/10 bell size is 24 kg, two bell sizes up is the 32 kg.

6 – KETTLEBELL CONDITIONING COMPLEXES

The last thing I'll mention is a kettlebell conditioning complex. Kettlebell complexes are outstanding for strength and conditioning. And, there are many options.

A COMPLEX IS A SERIES OF EXERCISES PERFORMED SEQUENTIALLY WITHOUT REST. ALL REPS OF ONE EXERCISE ARE COMPLETED BEFORE MOVING ON TO THE NEXT.

For example, here's a simple 3-exercise complex.

- kettlebell cleans x 5 reps right
- kettlebell cleans x 5 reps left
- kettlebell press x 5 reps right
- kettlebell press x 5 reps left
- kettlebell racked squat x 5 reps right
- kettlebell racked squat x 5 reps left

As you can see, that's 30 total reps with the kettlebell.

The complex is performed with one moderate-weight kettlebell and moving from exercise to exercise without rest.

The complex exercise combinations are limitless.

Very challenging, excellent for conditioning, and they will tax all 3 of your energy systems (Chapter 3).

There are many hormonal and metabolic benefits that occur when performing complexes because they involve a high level of work in a short period of time.

Complexes are great for:

- Conditioning
- Fat loss
- Lean muscle building
- General strength
- Mental toughness
- Stresses multiple energy systems

How many you do depends on your current conditioning level, but a good start point is 3 to 5 rounds with this complex.

APPROACHES TO CONDITIONING

There are many ways to approach conditioning.

The previous six examples are some of my favorites. Yet, I should also mention that I use specific interval and density training approaches, as well.

INTERVAL TRAINING

Interval training is performing an exercise for a given time period, followed by a specific rest period, and repeating the sequence for a specific number of rounds.

A fantastic interval training session is this simple swing workout. Here's how it works:

Set a timer for 30-second intervals. Every 30 seconds, perform one set of the following number of swings. Do these in order:

- 5 swings
- 10 swings
- 15 swings
- 20 swings

You can see that the rest time will decrease for each ascending set you do. After the final set of 20, rest a FULL 30 seconds, and then start over.

Do this for 10 minutes, so it's 4 rounds of ascending kettlebell swings.

I originally found this particular swing session from the great work by Tracy Reifkind.

To progress, use a heavier bell or add another round.

DENSITY TRAINING

Density training is about volume of exercise in a given time period. This is a way to progress your training in a specific time period.

The caution with density training is making sure you keep good technique and don't get sloppy.

There are multiple methods and ways to approach conditioning. As long as you're challenging your stamina, there's no wrong way to condition. Understand how the method you choose matches into your specific goals.

One of the easiest examples of a density session is the kettlebell snatch test.

A kettlebell snatch test is performing 100 kettlebell snatches in 5 minutes or less, and you can switch hands as many times as you need.

SNATCH TEST = 100 REPS IN 5 MINUTES OR LESS.

Men typically use a 24 kg kettlebell, while women use a 12 to 16 kg kettlebell depending on bodyweight.

One of the ways I like to approach the kettlebell snatch test is with a descending rep ladder. Here's what it looks like:

- 10 Right / 10 Left
- 9 R / 9 L
- 8 R / 8 L
- 7 R / 7 L
- 6 R / 6 L
- 5 R / 5 L
- 5 R / 5 L

The **psychological benefit** of performing a descending snatch test like this is amazing.

And, if you need to take a short break after 7 or 6, you can set the bell down briefly to catch your breath before beginning again.

I discovered this great protocol through my friend Betsy Middleton-Collie.

FAT LOSS, METABOLISM, AND STRENGTH

There's a large body of evidence to demonstrate that strength training has a major impact on our metabolism.

Remember, EPOC (or excess post-exercise oxygen consumption) from Chapter 3 – Important Terms and Concepts?

EPOC is the elevation of your metabolism AFTER exercise, which is a different effect from slow duration, traditional "cardio" training.

This is not to say that slow cardio training is ineffective for fat loss and metabolic effects; it's just much different.

If I'm going to do low-level cardio, then my preference is to go for long, fast paced walks. There are many benefits to adding a **"walking program"** into a strength-training approach.

There are benefits from strength training (as a whole) on our metabolism, not to mention to stimulation of important hormones such as **testosterone** and **growth hormone.**

Because of EPOC, the impact is improved fat-burning effects from the elevation of our metabolism.

I think there is a complete misunderstanding that many people have about the role of strength training for fat loss and the improvement of body composition.

But, **if you understand EPOC, you understand the significance of strength on our metabolism** to promote fat loss and to radically improve body composition.

This is why I prefer the combination of strength training and conditioning as opposed to long, slow cardio training.

CHAPTER 26: FUNCTIONAL HYPERTROPHY TRAINING

"Volume is the #1 driving force behind muscular hypertrophy."
–Dr. Brad Schoenfeld

I used to spend hours in the gym.

Back at the peak of my bodybuilding days, I was in the gym for 4 hours a day, 6 days a week.

While I don't advocate that much training and think it's excessive, the driving factor that worked for me at that time was the high volume.

To build muscle, you need to do more volume.

In Chapter 5, we discussed sarcopenia and the devastating consequences of muscle loss.

We need muscle.

This chapter will discuss how to build it.

In general, I've seen reports of muscle loss of 1% per year after the age of 40. And, that muscle loss begins around the age of 25 or 30 for most people.

I talked about how we lose muscle each year and how we want to do everything we can to prevent muscle loss.

Training for hypertrophy (or muscle building) has been a passion of mine for decades. But, it's not about aesthetics alone. Hypertrophy training should be a major goal for many of us because of the law of muscle loss.

Building muscle is challenging, but it's easier if we follow certain training principles.

To really pack on mass, you've got to eat a lot of food.

No, I mean, you have to eat A LOT of food.

There is a difference between adding quality lean muscle and packing on mass, so you have to be really clear on what your primary training goal is and train and eat appropriately for that goal.

The bottom line? It's lift heavy weight and do lots of reps.

The difference here is we are not talking about maximum loads like we'd use with powerlifting or even OL.

But, you're not using light weights either.

And, the way I like to work on muscle building today is much more functional than back when I was competing.

If you remember **myofibrillar hypertrophy** (denser, functional muscle) compared to sarcoplasmic hypertrophy (an increase in muscle cell volume), my approach is more designed to build myofibrillar hypertrophy.

For hypertrophy phases, I typically use:

- The big barbell lifts plus some free-form "bodybuilding" exercises
- Increased volume
- Progressive overload
- Specific hypertrophy principles
- A more "functional" approach versus my previous "bodybuilding" style

I will also use double kettlebell programs for hypertrophy, which have been very effective for me. If I don't use barbell program, a double kettlebell mesocycle is a great programming method for myofibrillar hypertrophy.

Let's talk about some of the key variables for hypertrophy, regardless of the tool you choose.

KEY DRIVERS FOR HYPERTROPHY

VOLUME

Volume can be defined as total reps, sets, and load.

Higher volume, multi-set programs have consistently produced the best gains with regards to hypertrophy.

INTENSITY

Intensity (as expressed as a percentage of 1RM) is also another significant training variable.

Loads of less than 65% 1RM are not sufficient to induce hypertrophy.

REPS

Rep ranges for hypertrophy are typically in the ranges of 8 to 12.

SETS

Sets per exercise are typically in the range of 3 to 5.

EXERCISES

This is dependent on whether large muscle groups are trained or smaller groups, but typically performed with 3 to 5 exercises per muscle group.

TIME UNDER TENSION

Time under tension (the time the muscle is spent under load) which increases muscle protein synthesis is another key driver to build muscle.

This is one reason why double kettlebell complexes are great for hypertrophy.

EXERCISE SELECTION

The highest value exercises are the multi-joint exercises, which recruit the most muscle fibers, although single-joint targeted exercises (e.g., biceps curls, triceps extension) are also useful and valuable in muscle-building programming.

MUSCULAR FAILURE

For the benefit of hypertrophy, training to muscular failure has been shown to be effective. However, this must be used with caution and should not be done for extended periods of time.

Training to failure for strength is not advisable, so keep the primary training goal in mind.

KEYS TO HYPERTROPHY TRAINING

If building muscle is the goal, the training variables need to be manipulated to meet the training goal.

Key considerations for hypertrophy programming:

- Rep ranges are typically between 8 to 12
- Rest intervals of 60 to 90 seconds between sets
- Multiple sets superior to single sets
- Multi-joint exercises and single-joint exercises
- Slower tempo on eccentric contraction
- Muscle failure techniques can be implemented, but with caution
- Hypertrophy phases should culminate with a taper phase to avoid overreaching

One of my favorite functional muscle-building programs is called **Barbell Bodybuilding,** which is a 6-week training cycle I built around the big barbell lifts.

The difference with my training today compared to years ago is that all the programming I do now is focused on functional improvement and improving my skills, even if body composition or aesthetics are a primary training goal.

Learn more about the powerful Barbell Bodybuilding program at RdellaTraining.com.

KETTLEBELLS FOR SIZE AND STRENGTH?

Absolutely.

The best way to gain size and strength with kettlebells is with a pair kettlebells, not just one.

Double kettlebells are twice the load and twice the impact.

Let's be clear, though; this is not bodybuilding. Bodybuilding is a specific way to train, and you most likely will not look like a bodybuilder training with kettlebells.

Instead, you can put on dense, functional muscle with a pair of kettlebells using the double kettlebell complex.

Kettlebells are appropriate for size and strength. And, heavy double complexes are the way to go here.

A simple example of a double kettlebell complex is a clean and press.

- 5 double kettlebell cleans
- 5 double kettlebell presses

One of the unique features of the complex is increasing time under tension which has been attributed to stimulating muscular hypertrophy.

And, double kettlebell complexes are extremely time-efficient training sessions.

Here are two great training resources and complete training programs for muscle-building using double kettlebell complexes:

- **The Shock and Awe Protocol** (RdellaTraining.com)
- **Kettlebell Muscle** by Geoff Neupert

Functional hypertrophy training is simply training for muscular development with an emphasis on also improving function, skill, and performance.

Who wouldn't want that?

CHAPTER 27:
PROGRAMMING MADE SIMPLE

"If you spend too much time thinking about a thing,
you'll never get it done."
–Bruce Lee

How do you get the best results from your training?

Programming.

For the final piece of *The Edge of Strength*, we'll discuss the importance of programming to maximize performance and results.

We've talked a lot about programming already. We've covered the concept of periodization, but now we'll dig deeper.

Proper programming is where great things happen – not good things, but great things.

Successful programming is how we get great results.

Great programming is all about the principles behind it, such as overload, specificity, and individualization. These are the key training principles. When we live by them, we'll continue to have success.

There are many great training programs for specific training goals.

I think programming is where people get hung up.

All you need to make programming easy, however, is this formula.

Pick the program that best matches your big goal, and do the program from start to finish.

In other words, train with purpose.

Great programs are built on specific principles – those are **the 7 laws** from Chapter 8. That's what great programming is built on.

Getting the best results (in anything) requires following a plan. We do agree on that, right?

A plan in training is referred to as "periodization" or a periodized approach. Before we discuss periodization more, we need to cover some differences in training approaches.

The way I see this is there are basically 3 major areas of how we approach training. Let's take them one by one.

RANDOMIZATION

First of all, **we do need variety.**

But, when there's no method to the madness, this is a problem. Not just a problem, but a major problem.

In my experience, randomization or random training, has consistently produced the worst results. As a matter fact, I've often said that random training produces random results if ANY results at all.

Unfortunately, this is the way most people train and wonder why no progress is being made.

On the other hand, there are certain aggressive programs (maybe you've seen some of those TV infomercials) they may produce results, but the question is – how has it actually made you better?

It should fit into your long-term plan, so always think long-term, not quick fix.

Most importantly, **does the program do anything to make you better and improve your movement and performance skills?**

For me, one of the worst outcomes I could think of would to be in the same spot 6 months from now.

12 months from now.

When I look at where I am today, as I write this, there are movements and skills I have significantly improved as compared to 6 months ago or a year ago. Olympic weightlifting is a specific example.

But, it my down years, I stayed the same and even regressed over time. I never really got better.

Why?

Lack of priority was a big reason, not to mention **lack of effective programming.** There were several reasons for this, but one was random training – not following a periodized approach or structured program.

Random training is going to the gym few times a week and doing what you feel like.

It's when you say, "I think today I'll do squats and presses. Tomorrow I'll do arms and back, maybe some abs. I'll do a few sets of this and maybe a few sets of that, then some cardio to finish off."

Maybe it's going to local big box gyms and following whatever the workout is that day. It's going through the motions, but not necessarily strategic or thoughtful training.

Random training is training with no plan, no method, no system.

It's training to "get fit" and "get in better shape." Listen, we all want to be fit and we all want to be in better shape, but **what does that mean?**

We have to quantify our fitness in some way. For more on how to clarify your goals, refer back to Chapter 17 – Finding Purpose.

Random training is a path that leads to the dreaded plateau, although there are frameworks to follow.

FRAMEWORK

A framework is simply following a set of principles that will provide a template for your training.

In contrast to periodization, which is a specific plan, a framework is a set of guiding principles. **A framework is a more loosely based program or template for training.**

It's a blueprint, but not necessarily as specific as a structured periodized approach, which we'll talk about soon.

Here's an example of a framework:

A 3 x 3 program can be used as a framework in your training.

The goal with the 3 x 3 is to improve strength.

Let's assume you have identified the exercises that you want to get stronger with (squat and deadlift, as examples).

Well, you simply follow the 3 x 3 training approach for the next 2 to 6 weeks.

You might be thinking, isn't this a structured program or a "periodized approach?"

Yes and no.

It is because you're following the 3 x 3 framework, but beyond the 2 exercises where you are doing a 3 x 3, you'd have freedom to add variety to your training.

In other words, with the 2 exercises (the squat and deadlift), you are following a more structured approach (the 3 x 3), but you have more freedom and flexibility as compared to a more structured program or plan.

You're following a framework to work toward specific goals, but it's NOT a fully structured program.

Don't get too hung up in this, just know that the framework is a **loosely based program that allows for more flexibility and variety, but it provides more structure than random training** (which has none).

I wouldn't suggest being completely random with the other exercises, but, narrow your options of exercises and make sure they contribute to your goals.

Your framework is the 3 x 3 with the two specific exercises, and then you have other exercises for variety. Yes, we do need variety and most people want variety. You're following a plan for some of what you do, but you also have the ability to choose other exercises based on how you feel on your training days.

Those other exercises could be for conditioning, for muscle building, or for whatever best aligns with the goals you identify.

I do frameworks in between structured programs or sometimes as "deloads," which we'll talk about soon.

The bottom line is that a framework is a loosely based program or system, it's NOT complete randomization. We can't follow programs all the time and that's where "framework" training comes into play.

PERIODIZATION

Periodization is defined as a sensible and well-planned approach to training that maximizes performance for specific goals.

It's the purposeful sequencing of different training variables for the desired state and results.

Periodization is a scientific concept developed during the 1950s through the 1970s in the former USSR by Russian scientists Matveyev, Ozlin, and others.

Periodization is a structured plan over an extended period of time.

This method is by far the most effective system for producing results, achieving peak performance, and accomplishing specific outcomes.

The extent that you use it will be determined by your goals and your commitment to plan, both in the short term and long term.

There are challenges to periodized approaches, and I understand that life keeps us all busy. Periodized approaches are much easier to follow for competitive athletes who are training specifically for an event like a competition.

Competitive athletes are role models for our success. Athletes are all about results, period. Winning is the end game. The most successful athletes, the ones who win, follow impeccable plans.

If we want success with our training, we can simply model what they do and follow a periodized approach.

A periodized approach may not be appropriate for everyone all throughout the year, but I can tell you **the more you plan, the more successful you will be in your training.**

Periodization is the ultimate strategy for both short-term and long-term planning.

TIMEFRAMES IN PERIODIZATION

In a periodized approach, program timeframes are broken down into microcycles, mesocycles, and macrocycles.

MICRO: 1 Week

Microcycles are typically a week of training or less.

MESO: 2 to 6 Weeks

Mesocycles are a number of weeks, typically 2 to 6 weeks in duration. A 6-week training program is an example of a mesocycle.

Most people will use the mesocycle for shorter term training success. There are many mesocycle programs for you to consider.

I'm a big fan of 4-to-6 week programs, then short periods of de-loading (a few days to one week). Some of the proven programs on **RdellaTraining.com** include:

- **The Shock And Awe Protocol** (4-week Strength and Hypertrophy Training)
- **Kettlebell Domination** (5-week Conditioning and Performance Program)
- **Barbell Bodybuilding** (6-week Functional Hypertrophy Training Program)

MACRO: 1 Year

Macrocycles are the annual training plan the typically involves peaking once a year at the time of the competitive event.

But, anyone can think big and think long term.

What if we planned our training for the long term instead of week to week or month to month?

Here's a simple way to apply the periodization concept to a macrocycle approach.

This is an example of a year long training plan into 4 distinct phases:

- 1st Quarter: Hypertrophy Phase
- 2nd Quarter: Strength Phase
- 3rd Quarter: Peaking Phase
- 4th Quarter: Performance/Technique Phase

Here you have an entire annual training plan to focus on for different goals, one goal at a time.

Another long term example over several months could be something like this:

- 8 weeks: General Prep Phase
- 8 weeks: Max Strength Phase
- 4-6 weeks: Conditioning Phase
- 8 weeks: Hypertrophy Phase

This is the approach that was essentially designed by Dr. Brad Schoenfeld in his book *The Max Muscle Plan*.

There are 2 keys to this long term approach, which we've discussed.

1. **Know your top goal.**
2. **Follow a specific plan to meet that goal.**

We've covered periodization. Next, let's discuss specific training variables.

REPS

Ok, let's review some important basic training concepts – reps and sets. For whatever reason, reps seem to be misunderstood, so let's cover the fundamentals.

The easiest way to think about reps with your training is as follows:

MAX STRENGTH ZONE: REPS OF 1 TO 3

Low-rep training with heavy weight is what leads to the most strength gains.

However, we have to be careful not to overtrain (or overreach). Typically it's only recommended to train low-rep ranges for short time periods.

Rep ranges in the max strength zone, as the name implies, will produce maximum strength development. However, this also taxes the nervous system to the extreme, so we need to be careful training in this zone and not train here for extended periods of time.

THE STRENGTH ZONE: REPS OF 4 TO 6

Repetitions between 4 and 6 are excellent for building strength, and the classic 5 x 5 program is a great example of a strength-producing system.

What we're doing in this rep range is using heavy enough yet reasonable weight to produce volume, which also is effective in producing muscular hypertrophy.

That's why the 5 x 5 program has been so effective for so many. It allows us to develop strength, and the volume benefits us by way of muscular hypertrophy.

HYPERTROPHY ZONE: REPS OF 8 TO 12

Typically, rep ranges between 8 to 12 are used for muscle building. This is the classic bodybuilding style approach.

In my bodybuilding days, this was the rep range I primarily trained for many years, keeping in mind my goal was only to build muscle.

Can you get strong training with rep ranges of 8 to 12?

Yes, providing you're training with heavy loads in those rep ranges, but this is not ideal for maximum strength or qualities of upper end strength. These rep ranges are clearly most effective for hypertrophy training – increasing the size of muscle fibers.

How you train and the variables you use completely depend on the training goal.

So if your goals are building muscle mass (hypertrophy) then this is where you want to be for a specified period of time. A mistake I made was always keeping things the same and not re-adjusting variables and establishing new goals.

STRENGTH ENDURANCE ZONE: REPS GREATER THAN 12

Strength endurance is performing strength-related activities over a longer period of time. When we're training in ranges of 12 reps and higher, clearly we're in the strength endurance zone.

A great example of strength endurance exercises are things like kettlebell swings and kettlebell snatches, in which both of these can be performed for high-volume and high repetitions.

Kettlebell swings and snatches are excellent demonstrations of strength endurance and work other attributes as well.

Higher volume work, typically over 12 repetitions, is most beneficial for improving the quality of strength endurance. Higher volume work with high repetitions is obviously also important for conditioning and fat loss programming.

SETS

As with everything else we've discussed, the number of sets you do is related to your goal and the peaking strategy.

More sets demand more energy and will take a lot more out of you, whereas doing fewer sets will be less demanding, take less time, and can yield potentially better results in terms of strength.

In general, **2 to 5 sets** is often used in many strength training regimens, but again this depends on the goal of the program and where the athlete is in their training cycle.

If an athlete is performing singles or doubles (1 or 2 reps), they may be doing 8 to 10 sets. So again, the variables will change depending on repetitions and many other important training considerations.

For strength-training purposes, many have success with 2 sets of 5 in a given exercise and progressively building volume up to the classic 5 x 5 approach.

If you're training for strength, never feel like 2 sets of 5 is not enough because it can be very effective – at least for a little while. Remember the important principle of progressive overload.

THE "3 TO 5" TEMPLATE – A FRAMEWORK

The "3 to 5" template is a simple training framework I use when not doing fully structured programs. The "3 to 5" template is a **framework** structured like this:

- 3 to 5 exercises
- 3 to 5 reps
- 3 to 5 sets
- 3 to 5 days per week
- 3 to 5 weeks

These are the simple guidelines for you to use in this framework program.

All of these training variables work extremely well for developing strength.

As we've covered, strength-training exercises do need to be progressed in an organized methodology (progressive overload, for example).

Let's cover the specifics of "3 to 5" so you can see how to put it all together.

EXERCISES

Pick 3 to 5 key exercises you want to focus on, most likely exercises from this book.

But they can be the key exercises that are most important for your identified goal or goals.

These 3 to 5 exercises will be the foundation for your program.

Example:

- **Barbell Back Squat**
- **Deadlift**
- **Press**
- **Kettlebell Swing**
- **Turkish Get-Up**

The exercises you choose are the focus, but you'll have the opportunity to do some other exercises as well.

I would even take this a step further and set one major exercise to focus on. Choose 5 exercises as the framework for your program, but ONE will be the primary area of focus.

In other words, if your big goal is to squat more, then squat more. By the way, I would recommend using a **training journal** to write down everything you do.

REPS

We'll keep reps in the range of 3 to 5. That's pretty simple.

The exception would be kettlebell swings or a similar conditioning exercise (e.g., kettlebell snatches, burpees, etc.).

Swings are typically done with higher reps for the benefits of conditioning, but the primary strength exercises (squat, press, DL) are to be done in the 3 to 5 rep range.

Do not exceed 15 reps total for any of the big lifts; keep reps in between 9 and 15 for each session. This would be 3 x 3 (9 reps total), 5 x 3 (15 reps total), or any other similar rep/set scheme. Just don't vary the total volume too much (ex. 5 x 5) with this framework.

SETS

All sets are 3 to 5, depending on how you feel and how you structure the program.

For example, one day you may want to perform only 3 sets of squats because you aren't "feeling it" that day.

Or maybe it's built in as a light day, while another day is set aside as a 5-set day with reps at 3 (15 total reps).

The point is that all sets are kept between 3 to 5 for the duration of this program.

FREQUENCY

Train 3 to 5 days per week.

I'd suggest determining how many days per week you'll train before you start the program.

Don't wing it here. This is not random training.

Plan it out or structure the frequency of the program before you start, either 3 days or 5 days.

I'll give you an example of what this looks like in just a minute.

DURATION

Do the "3 to 5" template for 3 to 5 weeks, no longer.

At the end of 3 to 5 weeks, de-load if you need to, and then **repeat or move on to something else.**

If you do go as short as 3 weeks, you could:

- Reassess and decide if you should continue to progress (most likely scenario)
- Take a few days to "de-load" if you feel you need to, then resume and progress for the second 3-week training block.

When you put together a program and sequence, always know why. What is the rationale behind the program and what you're doing?

Here's an example of the "3 to 5" template, based on a 3-day program for 3 weeks, using the 5 example exercises that I mentioned earlier.

DAY 1 (Mon)

- Deadlift, 3 x 3 at 80–85% 1RM
- Press, 3 x 3, work up to "heavy, but comfortable" 3 RM on last set
- Kettlebell Swings, 3 sets of 10–20
- Turkish Get Up, 3 reps per side
- Pull ups 2–3 sets of 5 (secondary, variety)

DAY 2 (Weds)

- Back Squat, 5 x 3, 80–85% intensity
- TGU x 3
- Push Press (variety press), 5 x 3
- Ab Wheel x 20 x 3
- KB Swings x 20 x 3

DAY 3 (Fri)

- Same as Day 1

DAY 4 (Mon)

- Same as Day 2. Since it's a new week, increase intensity or volume dependent on how you feel that day.

The key is to go slow, apply the principle of **progressive overload,** and keep all work in between the "3 to 5" guidelines (except for conditioning or supplemental exercises).

There is freedom and flexibility with this. It is based on rep and set schemes, but progression goes according to how you feel on the given training day. Don't over complicate this and just stick to the "3 to 5" guidelines I've outlined. It's simple and effective.

THE 5 X 5 SOLUTION – A PROVEN PROGRAM

"Save your strength for the next set."
–Alexander Faleev

The 5 x 5 method has been around for a long time because it's a program that works. **It's a simple solution for size and strength.**

Keep in mind, there are many different variations of the program.

The classic 5 x 5 is credited to the legendary bodybuilder and strongman Reg Park. If you aren't familiar with Reg, he had a 500-pound bench press as a bodybuilder.

Without question, the 5x5 is one of the most proven and battle-tested programs.

Mark Rippetoe, Mike Mahler, Bill Starr, Arnold and many others have used variations of the program for years.

Remember, the goal of the 5 x 5 is size and strength.

You should also understand that it is very demanding, depending on your **"training age"** (novice or advanced).

Ideally, the program is done with a barbell, but certainly it could be done with kettlebells, bodyweight training, or other training implements.

HOW I'VE USED THE 5 x 5

Pick 2 to 4 big lifts for the program.

My lift preferences are:

- **Squat**
- **Deadlift**
- **Bench press**

- **Military press**

These 4 lifts work perfectly for a 3 or 4 day a week program.

Find the weight that you can perform at least 2 strong sets of 5 with for each exercise.

This may be your approximate 7 RM weight.

Why?

Because you will do 2 "strong" sets, not 2 max sets.

The basic program is 6 weeks, adding a rep each week to work up to 5 sets of 5 in Week 6.

Let's take a look at the program, so you can see what I mean.

THE 5 X 5 PROGRAM TEMPLATE

This represents the reps for each workout during each week.

The goal is to work up to 5 x 5 in the 6th and final week before a de-load.

Week 1: 5, 5, 4, 3, 3

Week 2: 5, 5, 4, 4, 3

Week 3: 5, 5, 4, 4, 4

Week 4: 5, 5, 5, 4, 4

Week 5: 5, 5, 5, 5, 4

Week 6: 5, 5, 5, 5, 5

Week 7: DE-LOAD at 80% of previous weight

Week 8: RESTART with weight increased 2–5% of previous 5 RM.

WEEK 1 EXAMPLE

Day 1 (Monday) (WORKOUT A)

- Deadlift 5 RM weight x 5, x 5, x 4, x 3, x 3
- Military press 5 RM weight x 5, x 5, x 4, x 3, x 3

Supplemental exercises could be:

- Kettlebell swing x 15
- Pull-ups x 5
- Abs (ab wheel) x 20

Perform 3 sets of each.

Day 2 (Wednesday) (WORKOUT B)

- Squat 5 RM weight x 5, x 5, x 4, x 3, x 3

- Bench Press 5 RM weight x 5, x 5, x 4, x 3, x 3

Supplemental exercises:

- Good morning x 10 x 3
- Pull-ups x 5 x 2
- KB carry

Day 3 (Friday) *Light day @ 75% of the 5x5 day from previous

- Deadlift 5 RM weight x 5 reps, 4 sets
- Military press 5 RM weight x 5 reps, 4 sets

Accessory/tertiary exercises:

- Kettlebell swing x 15
- Pull-ups x 5
- Abs x 20
- Complete 2 or 3 rounds.

WEEK 2:

Begin with workout B. Rep sequence is noted in the template: 5, 5, 4, 4, 3.

When doing the **2nd workout** of Workout B, I'd typically **reduce volume and intensity** to work on more explosive lifts and technique.

For further clarification, **the 2nd workout** (the repeated exercises) **that week was always a lighter session,** so one is hard (the 5x5 session) and the other was a reduced-volume intensity session.

SUMMARY OF THE 5 X 5

The 5 x 5 program has many variations.

This is the variation I have used, which is based on 3 days of training.

The goal is to work up to 5 strong sets of 5 at the end of 6 weeks with the big lifts. You are gradually increasing volume over the 6 week time period.

This is a program that can be used over and over again, after appropriate periods of de-loading.

When you begin another 6-week block, the goal is to increase weight by 2 to 5%, dependent on training background.

Remember, if you're more of a novice, your gains will be far greater than the advanced lifter.

GET THE MOST OUT OF ANY PROGRAM

There are endless programs out there. Any great program follows the proven principles, which you can now reference at your convenience using this book.

Training programs depend on many factors and your programming needs to consider are based on whether you are:

- **novice**
- **intermediate**
- **advanced**

If you happen to remember Law #7 from Chapter 8, the GAS principle and the stages of alarm, resistance, and exhaustion, there will be big differences between how a novice responds versus an advanced athlete.

So, how do you find a program that's the best fit for you?

It's actually not difficult when you follow these steps.

STEP 1: THE ONE BIG GOAL

I've already discussed this in detail earlier, but this is where most mess up. It's really important to get clear.

This is the critical first step and also, it seems, the hardest. If you can get clear, you've got power and you're way ahead of most.

STEP 2: FIND A PROGRAM TO MATCH YOUR GOAL

There are many great programs available for strength, hypertrophy, conditioning, weightlifting performance, powerlifting, or whatever your primary goal is.

Pick one.

STEP 3: IMPLEMENT THE PROGRAM

Commit to the program when you start, and don't bail after a couple weeks because you don't think it's working for you.

You will learn what works and what doesn't, but you have to implement the program to find out.

One way or the other, you will have a result and discover a lot.

STEP 4: FINISH THE PROGRAM

And, finally . . .

There's a ton of programs.

Pick one and stick to it.

That's the secret, if there is one.

For more programming resources, here are a few books to check out. For more, please see the resources section at the end of the book.

- *Practical Programming for Strength Training,* 3rd Edition by Mark Rippetoe
- *5/3/1* by Jim Wendler
- *Easy Strength* by Pavel and Dan John
- *Deadlift Dynamite* by Andy Bolton
- *Power to the People* by Pavel
- *Simple and Sinister* by Pavel
- *Weightlifting Programming* by Bob Takano
- *Enter The Kettlebell* by Pavel

CONCLUSION

"Information without action is meaningless."
–Tony Robbins

There's a lot here, yet there's still so much to discuss.

The Edge of Strength attempted to cover the big picture in strength and performance.

I hope this book has had an impact on your approach to training for the long term.

I hope you've learned new things or gained a few key insights that will make a difference for you.

Remember, it's the little things that make a big difference.

I may not know you personally, but I really hope this book changed your life in a positive and meaningful way.

The Edge of Strength was written to help answer some very simple questions.

How can I get the best results from my training?

How can I make progress for the rest of my life?

And, how can I become the best version of myself to feel great, look great, and perform at the highest level?

This book attempted to approach those questions from as many angles as possible.

No doubt there is confusion, frustration, and misunderstanding about what to do to achieve extraordinary results in health and fitness.

Yet, the problem is already solved and always has been.

Focus on a foundation of strength.

As the great Olympic weightlifting champion, Tommy Kono, has said, "There is nothing new under the sun."

The big takeaway is simply this.

LIVE YOUR STRENGTH

That means living up to your potential and being the best version of you.

Being stronger makes life better.

The science has shown this, and I've shared with you my experiences through decades of training.

LIVE YOUR STRENGTH FOR THE REST OF YOUR LIFE

Something I touched on earlier in this book was the concept of training "for as a long as I am physically able."

What makes an individual STOP training?

This has been a burning question for me – why would someone stop training, knowing all the benefits that strength brings us?

I don't know if I'll be snatching a barbell at 90 years old, but I certainly may be deadlifting, at least on some level, for as long as I can safely perform a deadlift.

No matter who you are, how old you are, what your situation is, whether you consider yourself athletic or not, **it's never to late to live your strength**.

You and I were meant to be strong.

HONOR YOUR STRENGTH

We all have tremendous abilities and potential, but most people never even come close to what they have.

If you honor your strength, you'll move much closer to your potential.

Set big goals, aim high, and take bold action towards the things you want.

And, give back. Share what you learn and what you do with others. Help people. There are so many people who need our help so they can discover *The Edge of Strength*, as you have done.

Share your knowledge, help others become stronger, better versions of themselves. If you know people who need this book to understand the importance of the message, share it with them or recommend it to them.

We need to make the world stronger.

Strength is the most important physical quality we have because it helps so many other qualities and makes our lives better.

It not only improves our health and performance, but gives us an deniable edge in our lives.

Strength changes everything.

Now that this book has detailed the life-changing nature of strength, it's time to get strong and **become an unstoppable force.**

Focus on making progress each and every day. Live the 1% rule.

STRENGTH IS YOUR EDGE

The goal of this book was to help educate you on why strength is your edge for a better life.

It's the edge for greatness that lies inside each of us, regardless of age, gender, background, or experience.

I hope this guide has served you well on your quest to gain greater strength and be your best.

I hope one day we cross paths in our journey together.

Every day counts.

Every training sessions counts.

It's up to you . . .

LIVE YOUR STRENGTH.

DISCOVER YOUR GREATNESS.

REFERENCES AND CITATIONS

CHAPTER 1

- Arnold: The Education of a Bodybuilder by Arnold Schwarzenegger

CHAPTER 2

- The Way to Live by George Hackenschmidt
- Secrets of Strength by Earle Liederman
- The Development of Physical Power by Arthur Saxon
- Choose Yourself by James Altucher

CHAPTER 4

- Supertraining by Dr. Yuri Verkhoshansky and Mel Siff
- The Science and Practice of Strength Training by Dr. Vladimir Zatsiorsky and Dr. William Kraemer
- Advances in Functional Training by Mike Boyle
- **StartingStrength.com** by Mark Rippetoe
- **CatalystAthletics.com** by Greg Everett
- Intervention by Dan John

CHAPTER 5

- Sarcopenia: Burdens and Challenges for Public Health, Archives of Public Health, 2014

CHAPTER 6

- Power to the People by Pavel Tsatsouline
- Ruiz et al, Association Between Muscular Strength and Mortality in Men: Prospective Cohort Study, BMJ, July 2008, 337
- Larsson L, Grimby G, Karlsson J: Muscle strength and speed of movement in relation to age and muscle morphology. J Appl Physiol 1979, 46:451–456.

- Artero et al, A Prospective Study of Muscular Strength and All-cause Mortality in Men with Hypertension, J Am College Cardiol, 2011, May 3 57(18) 1831-1837

CHAPTER 7

- Movement by Gray Cook
- FunctionalMovement.com
- Barbosa Barreto de Brito et al, Ability to sit and rise from the floor as a predictor of all-cause mortality, Euro Jour of Prev Cardio, Dec 2012
- Born To Walk by James Earls
- What The Foot by Gary Ward

CHAPTER 8

- Power by Dr. Fred Hatfield
- Built to the Hilt by Josh Bryant

CHAPTER 9

- Human Anatomy and Physiology, Elaine Marieb, 1989
- J. Fisher et al., Evidence-Based Resistance Training Recommendations, Med Sport, 15 (3): 147-162, 2011
- K Koffer et al, Strength Training Accelerates Gastrointestinal Transit in Middle-aged and Older Men, Med Sci Sports Exercise, 1992 Apr;24(4):415-9.
- Fascia in Sport and Movement by Robert Schleip

CHAPTER 10

- The One Thing by Gary Keller and Jay Papasan

CHAPTER 11

- Original Strength by Tim Anderson and Geoff Neupert

CHAPTER 12

- Mastery by George Leonard

CHAPTER 15

- Death by Food Pyramid by Denise Minger

- It Starts With Food by Dallas and Melissa Hartwig
- Whole30.com
- M. Cornelis et al, Coffee, CYP1A2 Genotype, and Risk of Myocardial Infarction, JAMA, Vol. 295 No, 10, March 2006
- Primal Blueprint by Mark Sisson
- The Truth About Carbs by Nate Miyaki
- Fat Loss Happens On Monday by Josh Hillis and Dan John
- Nutrient Timing by Dr. John Ivey and Robert Portman
- ISSN Position Statement on Creatine

CHAPTER 16

- The Power of Less by Leo Babauta
- The Power of Habit by Charles Duhigg
- Your Bodies Many Cries For Water by F. Batmanghelidj
- Nutrition And Physical Degeneration by Weston Price
- Why Zebras Don't Have Ulcers by Robert Saplosky
- The Morning Miracle by Hal Elrod
- The Little Book of Talent by Daniele Coyle

CHAPTER 18

- The One Thing by Gary Keller and Jay Papasan
- Built to Last by Jim Collins

CHAPTER 19

- Eat That Frog by Brian Tracy

CHAPTER 20

- Your Body is Your Gym by Mark Lauren
- Convict Conditioning by Paul Wade
- Never Gymless by Ross Enamait
- Original Strength by Tim Anderson and Geoff Neupert
- Naked Warrior by Pavel

CHAPTER 22

- Enter The Kettlebell by Pavel

- Simple and Sinister by Pavel

CHAPTER 23

- Starting Strength by Mark Rippetoe
- Strong Enough by Mark Rippetoe

CHAPTER 24

- Olympic Weightlifting by Greg Everett
- Olympic Weightlifting for Sports by Greg Everett
- Encyclopedia of Olympic Weightlifting by Arthur Dreschler
- Championship Weightlifting by Tommy Kono
- Weightlifting Olympic Style by Tommy Kono

CHAPTER 25

- Ultimate MMA Conditioning by Joel Jamison

CHAPTER 26

- B Schoenfeld, The Mechanisms of Muscle Hypertrophy and Their Application To Resistance Training, J of Strength & Cond Research, Vol 24, No. 10, October 2010
- The Max Muscle Plan By Brad Schoenfeld

CHAPTER 27

- Practical Programming for Strength Training, 3rd Edition by Mark Rippetoe and Andy Baker
- 5/3/1 by Jim Wendler
- Easy Strength by Dan John and Pavel
- Deadlift Dynamite by Andy Bolton and Pavel
- Power to the People by Pavel
- Simple and Sinister by Pavel
- Enter The Kettlebell by Pavel
- Weightlifting Programming by Bob Takano
- The Max Muscle Plan by Brad Schoenfeld

ADDITIONAL RESOURCES

BOOKS

Recommended resources to further expand your learning of concepts discussed in this book.

GENERAL

- Never Let Go by Dan John
- Intervention by Dan John
- Can You Go by Dan John
- Before We Go by Dan John
  (Yes, Dan John has obviously been a major influence...)
- Ultimate Back Fitness and Performance by Stuart McGill
- The Power of Full Engagement by Jim Loehr and Tony Schwartz
- The Slight Edge by Jeff Olson
- Start With Why by Simon Sinek
- Live Life Aggressively by Mike Mahler
- Facts and Fallacies of Fitness by Mel Siff
- Make It Big by Frank McKinney
- The Encyclopedia of Underground Strength and Conditioning by Zach Even-Esh
- Mindless Eating by Brain Wansink
- Built to the Hilt by Josh Bryant
- The Way to Live by George Hackenschmidt
- Burn The Fat, Feed The Muscle by Tom Venuto
- The Purposeful Primitive by Marty Gallagher
- Strong Medicine by Chris Hardy and Marty Gallagher

MOVEMENT AND MOBILITY

- Movement by Gray Cook
- Supple Leopard by Kelly Starrett with Glen Cordoza
- Original Strength by Tim Anderson and Geoff Neupert
- What the Foot by Gary Ward

BODYWEIGHT TRAINING

- The Naked Warrior by Pavel Tsatsouline
- Your Body is Your Gym by Mark Lauren
- Never Gymless by Ross Enamait

- Convict Conditioning by Paul Wade

KETTLEBELL TRAINING

- Enter the Kettlebell by Pavel Tsatsouline
- Simple and Sinister by Pavel
- The Swing by Tracy Reifkind
- The Russian Kettlebell Challenge by Pavel

POWERLIFTING

- Starting Strength by Mark Rippetoe
- Practical Programming by Mark Rippetoe and Andy Baker
- 5/3/1 by Jim Wendler
- The Book of Methods by Louie Simmons
- Power To The People Professional by Pavel

OLYMPIC WEIGHTLIFTING

- Olympic Weightlifting by Greg Everett
- The Weightlifting Encyclopedia by Arthur Dreschler
- Olympic Weightlifting for Masters by Matt Foreman
- Bones of Iron by Matt Foreman

DVDS

- Kettlebells From the Ground Up DVD and Manual by Gray Cook and Brett Jones
- Dynami DVD and Training Manual by Gray Cook and Brett Jones
- Mastering The Hardstyle Kettlebell Swing by Mark and Tracy Reifkind
- Starting Strength DVD by Mark Rippetoe
- Olympic Weightlifting DVD by Greg Everett
- American Weightlifting – A Documentary

*These are just a few of the great continuing education resources from my personal library.

THE NEXT STEPS

The End?

No, this is only the beginning.

FREE RESOURCES FOR YOU

I always have FREE resources that are available at RdellaTraining.com to help people improve their training to get even better results.

Because I change things and update the FREE REPORTS and RESOURCES from time to time, the best way to see what's available is to go to:

RdellaTraining.com/join

You'll find the current gifts and valuable resources there, and you can join thousands of others who have become part of The Rdella Training community.

I'd also like to set up a special page for readers of this book to answer questions and expand concepts from *The Edge of Strength*.

Please visit **RdellaTraining.com/edgeofstrength**

SPREAD THE WORD

Your opinion and feedback matter.

If you benefited from this book and if this impacted you in a positive way, please do me a quick favor and drop in a review at Amazon.com.

I always say, if you take away just one big thing from any book you read and take action with it, it was worth your time.

That said, I hope that you took away several things from *The Edge of Strength* and take action with concepts and training approaches that I have shared with you.

And don't forget to share this book with friends, family, and your training buddies. I hope that this book ends up in the hands of many people to truly make a difference.

Your reviews make a difference, so help spread the word.

Thank you.

COACHING WITH SCOTT

Coaching and teaching is something I'm extremely passionate about. I appreciate the opportunity to work with people who want to get to the next level.

It's great to see people I work with make quantum leaps forward with their training and results.

As a **movement teacher** and **strength coach,** I'm committed to helping people discover what I have about how strength can improve all aspects of life.

There are opportunities for you and I to work together through my live seminars and online coaching where I will teach you the methods and techniques covered in this book.

Please check the pages below for more information.

- **RdellaTraining.com/coaching**
- **RdellaTraining.com/seminars**

PROGRAMS

SPECIFIC PROGRAMS

Available at RdellaTraining.com

THE SHOCK AND AWE PROTOCOL

The Shock and Awe Protocol is a 4-week double kettlebell program for the intermediate to advanced kettlebell enthusiast. The program is designed to build muscular hypertrophy and strength with double kettlebell complexes. It's a proven, powerful, time-efficient training cycle.

KETTLEBELL DOMINATION

Kettlebell Domination is 5-week single kettlebell program built on the fundamental exercises that are covered in this book. It is a progressive program designed to improve general strength and conditioning, as well as body composition. It's an intense program and requires experience with the kettlebell fundamentals.

BARBELL BODYBUILDING

Barbell Bodybuilding is a 6-week Functional Hypertrophy Training (FHT) program built around the barbell fundamentals, squats, deadlifts, and presses, as well as accessory exercises. This is a very effective program to build muscle mass and strength. This program requires experience with basic barbell lifts.

Go to **RdellaTraining.com/store** for the current programs and products.

To get the latest updates on **future programs and products,** go to...

RdellaTraining.com/join

ABOUT THE AUTHOR

Scott Iardella, MPT, CSCS, CISSN, SFGII, SFL, FMS, USAW, Pn1

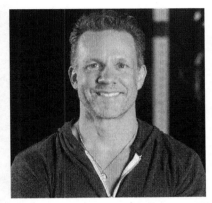

Scott Iardella is the Creator of **Rdella-Training.com**, an educational website dedicated to helping people of all backgrounds improve health and fitness through a foundation of strength.

Scott's focus is on performance with fundamental movements, kettlebells, and barbells to meet a wide variety of health and fitness goals.

Scott is a writer, coach, athlete, and host of **The Rdella Training® Podcast,** a leading weekly fitness podcast in iTunes.

With over 30 years of experience in the fitness and healthcare industries, Scott's background as a physical therapist, strength coach, and athlete offers unique perspective to bridge gaps in human performance.

Scott began his training journey as a teenager, and he competed in his first bodybuilding competition at the age of 19. He then competed for the next 6 years. The experiences of competitive bodybuilding and overcoming a major injury led him to obtain his Master's Degree in Physical Therapy from the University of Maryland.

Scott worked as an Orthopedic Sports Physical Therapist working with many amateur and professional athletes, as well as the general population. He specialized in shoulder, knee, and spine rehabilitation.

He is equally passionate about nutritional education to optimize health and performance and is a certified sports nutritionist.

Scott is certified by the National Strength and Conditioning Association as a Certified Strength and Conditioning Specialist. He is a Certified Sports Nutritionist by the International Society of Sports Nutrition, a Precision Nutrition, Level 1 Certified Fitness Professional, and a USA Level 1 Weightlifting Coach.

And finally, he is a certified kettlebell instructor who holds the StrongFirst Level II distinction, a StrongFirst certified barbell instructor and is also a Functional Movement Specialist.

For more learning and education about the methods and philosophy in this book, please refer to the links below:

- RdellaTraining.com
- Facebook.com/RdellaTraining
- Twitter.com/RdellaTraining
- YouTube.com/RdellaTraining
- Instagram.com/RdellaTraining
- The Rdella Training® Podcast in iTunes.
- Scientific Strength Podcast, also in iTunes

THANK YOU!

Thanks to you, the reader, for investing your time and energy into learning from this book.

Strength will bring you many rewards in your life for years to come – if you go about it the right way.

I hope you discover what I have through the material I have presented.

Thanks to...

Every client, patient, and individual I have ever worked with throughout the years. Those experiences have been invaluable.

Thanks to...

Just some of the outstanding professionals and mentors I've had the opportunity to work with and learn from in recent years – Pavel Tsatsouline, Dan John, Kelly Starrett, Gray Cook, Brett Jones, Andrea DuCane, Geoff Neupert, David Whitley, Jon Engum, Charlie Weingroff, Chad Wesley-Smith, Danny Camargo, Greg Everett, Glenn Pendlay, Travis Cooper, Mark Cheng, Mark Reifkind, Jeff O'Connor, Michael Hartle, Karen Smith, Betsy Middleton-Collie, Joe Sansalone, Kenneth Jay, and Dr. Jose Antonio and the ISSN. Special thanks to Frank McKinney.

I have been honored to continue to expand my knowledge from "world-class" leaders.

Thanks to...

Every outstanding guest that has graciously joined me on **The Rdella Training® Podcast** for the amazing conversations – Thank You!

Thanks to...

My family and friends for always supporting and encouraging me throughout my journey.

Train strong, train safe, and look for more to come!

Let me tell you something you already know...
The world ain't all sunshine and rainbows.
It's a very mean and nasty place, and I don't care how tough you are.
It will beat you to your knees and keep you there permanently –
if you let it.
You, me, or nobody is gonna hit as hard as life. But, it ain't about how
hard you hit, it's about how hard you can get hit –
AND KEEP MOVING FORWARD.
How much you can take and keep moving forward.
That's how winning is done.
You gotta be willing to take the hits.
–Rocky